Intermittent Fasting for Women Over 50

Successfully Lose Weight in 5 Steps to Transform Your Body, Restore Hormonal and Heart Health, Reduce Inflammation, and Strengthen Brain Function Without Dieting or Counting Calories

Erin Hanson

© Copyright 2022 - All rights reserved.

The content contained within this book may not be reproduced, duplicated or transmitted without direct written permission from the author or the publisher.

Under no circumstances will any blame or legal responsibility be held against the publisher, or author, for any damages, reparation, or monetary loss due to the information contained within this book, either directly or indirectly.

Legal Notice:

This book is copyright protected. It is only for personal use. You cannot amend, distribute, sell, use, quote or paraphrase any part, or the content within this book, without the consent of the author or publisher.

Disclaimer Notice:

Please note the information contained within this document is for educational and entertainment purposes only. All effort has been executed to present accurate, up to date, reliable, complete information. No warranties of any kind are declared or implied. Readers acknowledge that the author is not engaged in the rendering of legal, financial, medical or professional advice. The content within this book has been derived from various sources. Please consult a licensed professional before attempting any techniques outlined in this book.

By reading this document, the reader agrees that under no circumstances is the author responsible for any losses, direct or indirect, that are incurred as a result of the use of the information contained within this document, including, but not limited to, errors, omissions, or inaccuracies.

Table of Contents

INTRODUCTION 1

PART 1: WHAT IS INTERMITTENT FASTING? 5

CHAPTER 1: AN AGE-OLD TRADITION 7

THE HISTORY OF FASTING 7
   Religious Fasting 7
   Medical Fasting 8
   Fasting in the Modern Era 9
THE HISTORY OF DIETING 11
   1820: Vinegar and Water Diet 12
   1903: Fletcherism 12
   1920s: Cigarette Diet 13
   1930s: Hollywood Diet 13
   1961: Weight Watchers 13
   1970: Sleeping Beauty Diet 14
   1972: Nutrisystem 14
   1975: Paleo Diet 15
   1977: SlimFast 15
   1979: Pritikin 15
   1983: Jenny Craig 16
   1985: Fit for Life 17
   1992: Atkins 17
   1995: Zone Diet 18
   2003: South Beach Diet 18
   2009: Whole30 18
   2011: HCG 19

CHAPTER 2: INTERMITTENT FASTING AND WOMEN'S HEALTH . 21

THE IMPACT OF "THE CHANGE" 21
   Perimenopause 21
   Menopause and Postmenopause 23
THE CASE FOR IF 24

CHAPTER 3: FASTING METHODS...29

12:12 30
16:8 31
EAT STOP EAT 32
23/1 (OMAD) FASTING 33
2-DAY FAST 34

WEEKLY 24-HOUR FAST 34
MEAL SKIPPING 35
WARRIOR DIET 37

PART 2: HOW IF WORKS 39

CHAPTER 4: WHAT HAPPENS WHEN WE FAST 41

THE FED STATE—HOURS 0–4 41
THE EARLY FASTING STATE—HOURS 4–16 42
THE FASTING STATE—HOURS 16–24 44
ENTERING THE STARVATION STATE—HOURS 24–72 46
STARVATION—HOURS 72+ 47
ENDING A FAST 48

CHAPTER 5: UNDERSTANDING THE KEYS TO IF 51

SYSTEMS WORKING TOGETHER 52
THE METABOLIC SWITCH 54
AUTOPHAGY 57

PART 3: BENEFITS OF IF 61

CHAPTER 6: WEIGHT LOSS 63

REDUCED CALORIC INTAKE 63
REDUCED HUNGER 66
REPAIRED METABOLISM 68
INCREASED AUTOPHAGY 69
REPAIRED INSULIN RESISTANCE 69
OVERALL FINDINGS 70

CHAPTER 7: BRAIN AND MENTAL HEALTH 73

BRAIN HEALTH 73
Improvements in Overall Brain Function *74*
Protection Against Disease *76*
MENTAL HEALTH 77
Improved Mood *78*
Reduced Anxiety and Stress *79*
Reduced Depression *79*

CHAPTER 8: PROTECTION FROM INFECTION AND ILLNESS 81

COVID-19 81
THE IMMUNE SYSTEM CONNECTION 83
Fasting Regenerates Immune Cells *84*
Fasting Reduces Inflammation *84*
FASTING HELPS REDUCE CHRONIC PAIN 85
EFFECTS ON CANCER AND CANCER TREATMENT 86
Reduced Cancer Risk *87*
Reduced Side Effects of Chemotherapy and Radiation *88*

Insulin and IF.. *88*

CHAPTER 9: CELLULAR AND PHYSICAL GROWTH........................... 91

WHAT DOES FOOD ADDICTION HAVE TO DO WITH IT?...................................... 91
HEALTHY GROWTH 93
Increases in Stem Cells.. *93*
Mitochondria Repair... *94*
Improved Gut Health *95*
Increased Human Growth Hormone (HGH).. *97*
Decreased Androgen Markers in Women *98*

PART 4: HOW TO INTERMITTENT FAST 101

CHAPTER 10: MENTAL/PHYSICAL PREPARATION AND TRAINING
.... 103

ADJUST YOUR VIEW OF EATING.. 103
Develop a Good Relationship With Food *104*
Get a Good Night's Sleep.. *106*
Learn How to Recognize When You Are Hungry... *107*
Be Mindful About What You Are Eating *107*
Take Small Steps and Be Realistic About What You Can Do *108*
DON'T FORGET THE SUPPLEMENTS 108
PHYSICAL TRAINING TO ENHANCE YOUR RESULTS.. 111

CHAPTER 11: BUILDING A BALANCED DIET PLAN...........................115

HOW AND WHAT TO EAT... 115
Choosing the Right IF Protocol... *115*
Choosing the Right Foods to Eat.. *119*
MACROS… MICROS… HUH?... 121
Getting the Right Kinds of Fat.. *122*
Getting Enough Protein *123*
Getting the Right Amount of Carbs *124*

CHAPTER 12: POPULAR DIET PROGRAMS... 127

HIGH-PROTEIN DIET 128
LOW-CARB DIET... 128
LOW-FAT DIET 129
MEDITERRANEAN DIET 130
PALEO DIET 131
KETO DIET.. 132

PART 5: LIFESTYLE TRANSFORMATION.. 135

CHAPTER 13: TRANSFORMING YOU IN 5 STEPS: YOUR PATH AND YOUR PACE 5-STEP PROGRAM TO FINDING SUCCESS WITH IF 137

STEP 1: DECIDE ON YOUR DIET PLAN 138
STEP 2: CHOOSE THE FASTING METHOD TO START.. 138

Step 3: Select Your Starting Point 139
Step 4: Customize a 6-Week Program 139
Step 5: Maintain a 40-Day IF Schedule and Chart Your Success 140

CONCLUSION 141

GLOSSARY 143

REFERENCES 147

Introduction

Just believe in yourself. Even if you don't, pretend that you do, and at some point, you will. –Venus Williams

Weight snuck up on me. I bet you know what I mean.

One day, I was doing okay. I have never been skinny, but I was fit. I put on some weight in my twenties and thirties. But everybody does. I mean, looking like a movie star is a full-time job!

Gradually, though, none of the things I was doing to keep myself in shape and looking good seemed to work. I just kept gaining weight, and it made me feel bad about myself. My moods were all over the map. Sometimes sex was really uncomfortable. This all made me feel worse! And I wasn't even 45.

It was a shock to discover I had started menopause.

Yes, I knew "The Change" was coming... sometime in the future. Maybe when I was in my 50s? I knew that menopause meant that I would no longer get a period. I had heard of hot flashes and mood swings. But I had never heard the term perimenopause: those four years or so during which your ovaries gradually stop making eggs, and periods become irregular, before they finally stop.

It was when I was deep into the experience of perimenopause that I saw a poster with this quote from Venus Williams, and I took it to heart. I was reminded that life is difficult for everyone. What matters is what you do about it.

We always used to say "fake it until you make it." It was affirming to hear the same thing from someone so accomplished.

I knew I could find my way back to being me. I just needed to take control. My goal with this book is to share what I learned on that journey.

I am not a doctor and this is not a book of medical advice. It is always a good idea to consult a physician before making major diet or other lifestyle changes that affect your health. But I do want to share the experience of what worked for me, and what I have seen work for many of my friends.

And please be aware if you have an eating disorder, some of what you might read in this book may be a trigger for you. It is not my intention in any way to body-shame. Healthy people come in all shapes and sizes. My goal is to share how intermittent fasting helped me take healthy control of *my* diet and fitness.

Our bodies change as we get older. Most mature bodies do not look anything like we see in most movies, videos, and magazines.

The fact is, menopause is just one of the things that causes our bodies to change; but it is a big one, because menopause affects your hormonal balance and changes your metabolism. When extreme, these changes can actually put you at risk of chronic illness such as heart disease, cancer, sleep apnea, or Type 2 Diabetes ((Hormonal Weight Gain, 2022).

The result is that most women gain five to eight percent of their pre-menopausal body weight in the first two years (Boynton, 2022). So, a menopausal woman who is relatively fit and trim, perhaps 5'6" tall and weighing 130 lbs, will gain 6.5 lbs if everything else in her life stays the same.

You can see it in the numbers. The average 20–39-year-old woman in the US is 5'4" tall and weighs 168 lbs. The average woman age 40–59 weighs 176 lbs; and the average woman age 60 and older weighs 167 lbs (Marcin, 2017).

For many of us, the added weight of menopause is the tipping point of a progression of added pounds that accumulates gradually over the years.

One big cause of weight gain is pregnancy and the lifestyle changes related to raising children. Stress is another trigger, perhaps caused by work, divorce, financial problems, chronic illness, or emotional problems. Ironically, even dieting can be a cause of weight gain (we'll talk more about this later).

The first step to taking control is to accept the fact that, during and after menopause, we women need to change our lifestyle in order to maintain a healthy weight. We need to understand that it is about more than numbers on a scale; it is about pounds plus body fat and muscle mass.

Intermittent fasting (IF) turned out to be the key element of my new lifestyle, and I am not the only one.

An article in *People* listed nine stars and celebrities who have embraced IF (Cho, 2020):

- actresses Jennifer Aniston, Vanessa Hudgens, and Kate Walsh

- Twitter CEO Jack Dorsey

- actor Chris Pratt

- media personality Kourtney Kardashian

- singer Moby

- model Molly Sims

- talk-show host Jimmy Kimmel

At around the same time, *Marie Claire* published a similar list which also included:

- Gisele Bündchen, model and wife of the notoriously healthy Tom Brady

- actresses Halle Berry, Reese Witherspoon, Scarlett Johansson, Elsa Pataky (and her husband Chris Hemsworth), and Mindy Kaling

Importantly, in their interviews these folks talk about both how IF works for them as a diet and how it helps them to feel healthier.

In addition, there is a growing body of research reported in places like the *Journal of American Medicine (JAMA) Network Open* and the *Annual Review of Nutrition* that shows the overall benefits of intermittent fasting, and that IF can be a valuable part of a healthy diet and lifestyle for perimenopausal and menopausal women (Landau, 2022).

So, take the journey with me to learn how you can regain control of your diet, your fitness, confidence, inner discipline, and overall well-being.

Part 1:

What Is Intermittent Fasting?

Part 1:

What Is Intermittent Fasting?

Chapter 1:

An Age-Old Tradition

The discipline of fasting breaks you out of the world's routine. –Jentezen Franklin

Fasting is not the same as starving. To fast is to restrict food intake by choice, and it is a practice that has been around for millennia.

According to the Merriam-Webster dictionary, to fast is "to abstain from food," or "to eat sparingly or abstain from some foods." It is a discipline, and the very definition indicates the fact that a fasting discipline can be practiced in different ways.

The History of Fasting

Religious Fasting

I started this chapter with a quote from Jentezen Franklin. Franklin is an evangelical televangelist and the author of half a dozen books about fasting (Jentezen Franklin, 2022). He is just one exemplar of the relationship between fasting and religion.

Religion is a part of human society the world over. It is one the original cultural institutions. And some form of fasting is often an element of religious practice.

Christians fast during Lent. Muslims fast during Ramadan. Jews fast during Yom Kippur. In Native American societies, fasting is a component of the vision quest. It is practiced in various ways by Buddhists, Taoists, Hindus, and followers of Jainism.

The concept of fasting is a broad one. It ranges from refraining from certain foods to refraining from ingesting anything at all for a prescribed period of time. For example, Christians who observe the 40 days of Lent choose to refrain from certain foods, often something that they especially enjoy. To observe Yom Kippur, Jews refrain from all eating or drinking for 25 hours. During the month of Ramadan, Muslims refrain from eating or drinking from dawn to sunset. Monks and some other followers of Buddhism fast daily, eating only during the hours between sunrise and midday.

Journalist Dag Kättström, who covers biomedical research, diet, and health, has explored the development of fasting as a religious tradition. He writes that in prehistoric hunter–gatherer societies, where food was not always available, the practice of fasting may have been practiced by societal groups as a way to increase the group's chance of survival. By fasting, they preserved food for an uncertain future. Then, due to its importance, the practice of fasting was incorporated into religious tradition. It was embraced as a way to both practice sacrifice and focus the mind on important values.

Significantly, over the years, people who participate in religious fasting have reported positive short-term physical as well as spiritual effects. These include lowered cholesterol and decreased insulin resistance (Kättström, 2019).

Medical Fasting

This brings me to the second thread in the tradition of fasting: fasting for therapeutic reasons.

We come to therapeutic fasting instinctively.

Think about how you feel when you are sick. Do you want to eat? Probably not. This natural inclination to restrict, even abstain from, eating and drinking when you are sick can be seen as the body's way to heal.

According to the Encyclopedia Britannica, fasting for medical benefit has been prescribed since the time of the ancient Greeks. For example, we know that Hippocrates, the physician who lived c. 460–c. 375 BCE, recommended fasting to help cure some illnesses, as did his successors, including another foundational physician, Galen.

The practice continued. The 16th century physician Paracelsus wrote, "Fasting is the greatest remedy–the physician within" (Fung, 2015).

Starting in the 1800s, doctors and researchers started to study the effects and benefits of fasting. An article on the website *healthline* summarizes eight evidence-based ways fasting has been found to improve your health (Link, 2018):

- reduced insulin resistance

- decreased inflammation throughout the body

- improved levels of good cholesterol and blood pressure

- improved brain function

- increased metabolism and promoting weight loss

- increased levels of human growth hormone

- delayed effects of aging

- enhanced effects of chemotherapy and potential prevention of cancer

I'll go into more detail on these benefits in Part 3 of this book.

Fasting in the Modern Era

The German doctor Otto Buchinger (1878–1966) is credited as the first to develop the type of therapeutic fasting protocol that is followed today. Dr. Buchinger came to realize the benefits of fasting through personal experience. He suffered from severe rheumatism that made it hard for him to continue working, and he decided to treat himself by undergoing a 19-day fast. His protocol combined a very restricted diet (fruit and vegetable juice, vegetable broth, honey, and lots of fluids) with physical, mental, and spiritual therapies (Visioli et al., 2022).

Dr. Buchinger's fasting cure was successful. As a physician and scientist, he followed up by documenting the results of fasting, and in 1935 he published a book called *The Therapeutic Fasting Cure* which described its effects and benefits in detail. He recommended that fasting be medically supervised and opened several clinics which are still in operation today (History of Therapeutic Fasting - BUCHINGER WILHELMI, n.d.).

Physician Isaac Jennings and naturopath and chiropractor Herbert Shelton were major promoters of therapeutic fasting in the United States (Goldhamer et al., 2015). Their work places fasting in both the medical and natural, or alternative, medical traditions.

Dr. Jennings practiced medicine in Connecticut in the 1800s. He was one of the first doctors in the United States to recommend fasting as a cure for disease. Starting in 1822, Jennings began to prescribe fasting as part of a natural therapeutic treatment that also included eating a vegetarian diet, seeking emotional balance, and getting plenty of exercise water, sunshine, fresh air, and rest. Jennings' treatment came to be known as natural hygiene.

Jennings' work inspired a 20th century promoter of fasting: Herbert Shelton. Shelton developed a strict, water-only fasting program. He went on to help found the Natural Hygiene Society, dedicated to the promotion of a hygienic lifestyle that included fasting. In 1978 that organization established a professional branch called the International Association of Hygienic Physicians that studies fasting and certifies physicians who supervise fasting therapy.

In addition to these two medical approaches, another trend in the modern era has been the promotion of fasting simply as a way to lose weight. The reason for this can be seen in the history of agriculture and food production.

An article on the U.S. Chamber of Commerce website documents how modern agricultural productivity has brought much of the world out of a subsistence economy (Schulz, 2012). The resulting agricultural bounty put food on the shelves of stores around the world.

Unfortunately, the combination of this abundance with industrial food production, food product marketing, and increasingly sedentary lifestyles are among the causes of an epidemic of obesity. These are not the only factors, but they are easily seen and understood (McAllister et al., 2009). One result has been a focus on the idea of fasting—restricting food intake—as a straightforward way to lose weight.

Intermittent fasting, which focuses on when you eat as well as what you eat, is one way to do this. But before we explore the details of intermittent fasting, let's take a look at what may be a more familiar type of fasting: dieting.

The History of Dieting

Dieting is nothing new. But—as explained in an article in BBC News Magazine—the word *diet*, which derives from the Greek *diatia*, used to be more than what you ate. It referred to an entire healthy lifestyle. The idea of dieting for weight and beauty really began in the 19th century, and the craze for dieting inspired a host of patent medicine charlatans and some preposterous fad diets (Winterman, 2013).

One of the first fad diets was inspired by the poet Lord Byron, a major celebrity of his day, who drank vinegar and ate vinegar-soaked potatoes. An early 20th century fad was Fletcherism, also called chew and spit.

Let's examine these and other examples from the history of dieting.

1820: Vinegar and Water Diet

Lord Byron was one of the first celebrity fad diet advocates, but even though Byron's stringent dieting contributed to his early death, the idea of a vinegar and water diet still has some adherents.

In its modern incarnation, the idea is simply to consume healthy foods in moderation, exercise, and drink a small amount of vinegar water every day. The vinegar is combined with water to reduce acid damage to the enamel of your teeth.

There is research that suggests that apple cider vinegar can make you feel full and that a small daily amount of vinegar can reduce levels of glucose and cholesterol (Aurametrix, 2009). Even without drinking vinegar, though, we know that eating moderate amounts of healthy food and exercising regularly will help you achieve a healthy weight.

1903: Fletcherism

Fletcherism is named for its creator, Herbert Fletcher. The central idea of Fletcherism was to eat only when hungry, be aware of the nutritional value of what you eat, eat slowly, and stop eating when you are full. But the method prescribed for doing this went to the extreme (Djublonskopf, 2015).

Practitioners of Fletcherism believed in chewing each mouthful hundreds of times until the food became liquefied, and then spitting out what remained. You were even supposed to chew liquids in order to extract all flavor. You could tell that you were doing it right if you defecated seldom and the results were odorless.

The popularity of Fletcherism made Fletcher a millionaire. But the diet was wildly impractical, and taken to extremes not very healthy.

1920s: Cigarette Diet

This diet was actually created as part of an advertising campaign for the Lucky Strike brand of cigarettes. The idea was simple: When you are hungry, smoke a cigarette instead. The diet works. Nicotine does suppress your appetite. Unfortunately, it also causes cancer (Foley, 2018).

In fact, one of the challenges smokers face when they try to stop smoking is that they often gain weight.

1930s: Hollywood Diet

The Hollywood, or Grapefruit, Diet is said to have been created for the actress Ethel Barrymore. The idea was to consume just 800 calories a day for 18 days by eating nothing but half a grapefruit and such low-calorie foods as oranges, toast, vegetables, and eggs.

The Hollywood Diet is just one example of many restricted-calorie diets, an idea that was first made popular by physician Lulu Hunt Peters. Other examples include the cabbage diet, the cookie diet, and— most extreme— the Last Chance Diet, which actually caused deaths by restricting adherents to 400 calories a day from a special drink that was made from a combination of hides and other meat byproducts.

1961: Weight Watchers

Weight Watchers substitutes counting points for counting calories. Dieters keep a record of what they eat every day and try to eat foods that add up to just the recommended number of points.

The diet has evolved since it was introduced, and has been rebranded as WW (Wellness That Works). Unlike the original program, which limited both calories and the foods you were permitted to eat, the program today allows any food. It assigns points based on a combination of calories, overall nutritional value, and exercise rather than on calories alone.

WW is a commercial program. There is information available you can use to follow the Weight Watchers protocol for free, but if you choose to pay a monthly fee, programs range from a digital app to plans with group or even individual coaching.

1970: Sleeping Beauty Diet

The idea behind this diet is to eat less by sleeping more. The problem is, in order to do that you need to use sedatives so you can sleep as much as 15 hours each day, and both the continued use of sleeping pills or other sedatives and oversleeping are bad for you.

Among the detrimental effects of this diet are: memory loss, depression, and increased risk of diabetes or stroke. It is an indication of how unhealthy this diet is that the idea for it originated in the pro-anorexia community (Rana, 2018).

1972: Nutrisystem

Nutrisystem is another commercial diet program. It is a high-protein diet designed to keep blood sugar levels steady.

Dieters subscribe to a plan of prepackaged meals, supplemented by additional groceries. The program restricts calories by controlling content and portions. To start, dieters work with a counselor to select one of the company's meal plans. In week one, they eat only prepackaged Nutrisystem meals. Then in week two, they are coached to start cooking meals for themselves.

Various program levels include a mobile app, supplements, and coaching. However, because they are designed for weight loss, the Nutrisystem meals have fewer calories than recommended.

1975: Paleo Diet

The Paleo Diet is an attempt to align nutrition today with the diet of our prehistoric ancestors. It is based on the idea that, due to the slow pace of evolution, what was good for us then is best for us now.

Although the term "paleo" was not introduced until later, the diet was popularized by a book, *The Stone Age Diet*, written by gastroenterologist Walter Voegtlin. Voegtlin argued that humans can most easily digest natural animal fats, proteins, and roughage—not synthetic nutrients, bulking agents, and carbohydrates.

1977: SlimFast

SlimFast is another commercial diet program that markets a line of prepackaged meals, shakes, snacks, and meal bars. Its first product was a line of diet shakes intended to be eaten for breakfast and lunch. The program suggested limited calories at supper by using other prepackaged meals such as Lean Cuisine frozen dinners.

SlimFast is geared toward people who want to lose weight but have a hard time preparing nutritious, low-calorie meals for themselves. Because the SlimFast products are low in calories, people who use the program are able to lose weight. And the company even sells a line of products branded for intermittent fasting.

1979: Pritikin

The Pritikin diet calls for eating lots of whole grains and other dietary fiber, little cholesterol and fat, and less protein than normally suggested. It tells you how many servings from each of the various food groups to eat every day, and also recommends 45 minutes of moderate exercise a day. Another idea central to the Pritikin diet is to eat more food that is high in bulk but low in calories, which helps you feel full without overeating.

The Pritikin diet was developed by an engineer, Nathan Pritikin, who was diagnosed with heart disease at a time when the typical American diet was high in fat but standard treatments did not include dietary or lifestyle recommendations.

Pritikin created a heart-healthy diet, which became popular after he and his cardiologist appeared on the TV show *60 Minutes* to promote the diet's effectiveness. There is now a body of research that validates the Pritikin diet principles, which have been incorporated into medical recommendations for patients who have cardiovascular disease.

Pritikin is a relatively low-calorie diet, so people who follow the plan typically do lose weight; but the primary goal is cardiovascular health rather than weight loss. If a person follows the Pritikin plan for weight loss but then returns to earlier dietary habits, he or she will likely regain weight that was lost.

1983: Jenny Craig

Jenny Craig is another commercial weight-loss company with a program based on the sale of its food products. The program incorporates private coaching (in person or virtual), an activity plan geared to fit into your normal daily life, and intermittent fasting. There are three programs: the basic meal plan, an accelerated weight loss plan, and a special plan for people who have Type 2 diabetes.

Diets start at 1,200 calories per day, increasing to 2,300 calories per day. People who follow the program eat primarily Jenny Craig prepackaged meals until they are halfway to achieving their weight loss goal, after which the coach helps guide them to preparing their own meals to provide a daily calorie limit that will maintain the desired weight.

One of the features now incorporated into the Jenny Craig program is called Volumetrics, which mirrors the high-bulk/low-calorie recommendation of the Pritikin diet.

1985: Fit for Life

The Fit for Life program was created by a self-styled nutrition expert. The central concept is the idea that you lose weight based not on caloric intake but on the combinations of food that you eat.

Harvey and Marilyn Diamond, the founders of Fit for Life, are proponents of natural hygiene. They advocate eating "living foods" (raw vegetables and fruits) and avoiding "dead foods" (starch and meat). Its rules include eating only fruit and fruit juice in the morning, eating either vegetables or carbohydrates for lunch and dinner (but not both), never eating dairy or drinking water with a meal, and eating whatever you want one day a week.

It is possible to lose weight on Fit for Life, but because Fit for Life is not necessarily a well-balanced diet it can cause problems like calcium and other mineral or vitamin deficiency.

1992: Atkins

This diet was created by cardiologist Robert Atkins. The goal is to change your metabolism by minimizing carbohydrates and eating some protein along with foods that are high in fat. You do not have to worry about portion size or count calories. You only count carbohydrates. There are four phases to the diet, from the more restrictive weight loss plan to a less restrictive maintenance plan.

Carbohydrates provide energy for your body. Because excess sugar is stored in the body as fat, a diet low in carbohydrates will cause your body to burn that fat for energy.

Dieters avoid white bread (made with refined grains), cake and cookies, pasta, rice, and potatoes (including chips and fries). They eat lots of proteins, nuts, non-starchy vegetables, low-sugar fruits, and whole grains.

According to the Cleveland Clinic, this diet can work to control weight because you won't feel hungry even though the diet does cut calories. However, some people who follow the diet end up eating too much processed meat and too few types of fruits and vegetables. This can cause constipation or kidney problems. Also, when your body burns fat instead of sugar for fuel, you will experience ketosis, which causes bad breath.

1995: Zone Diet

This diet was developed by biochemist Barry Sears. Sears lost several family members to heart disease and wanted to create a diet that would reduce inflammation in the body.

Dieters eat 40% complex carbohydrates, 30% lean proteins, and 30% fat, consumed in three meals and two snacks.

The simplest way to follow this diet is to use a hand-eye method, which measures portions based on the size of your hand. A more rigorous plan is called Zone food blocks and is based on precise calculations of grams in the carbohydrates, proteins, and fats that you eat. How precise? A sample Zone block snack might specify one hard-boiled egg, three almonds and half an apple.

2003: South Beach Diet

This is a commercial diet created by a cardiologist, Arthur Agatston. It is modeled on the Atkins diet, although it has three rather than four phases, and it limits carbohydrates and fats. There is more focus on selecting the right carbohydrates for maximum weight loss. It also includes an exercise component. Dieters do their own cooking but purchase meal plans.

2009: Whole30

Whole30 is what is called an elimination diet, intended to be used for 30 days to achieve weight loss. It is similar to the Paleo diet, but has even more restrictions. The idea is to eat only meat and seafood, nuts and seeds, vegetables, fruit, and eggs. Dieters also avoid all sugar, dairy, legumes, grains, and alcohol.

2011: HCG

HCG, or human chorionic gonadotropin, is a hormone made during pregnancy and is also used medically as a fertility treatment. In 2011, the Food and Drug Administration (FDA) cracked down on homeopathic HCG supplements that were being sold as an appetite suppressant and weight loss aid (Hensley, 2011).

HGG diet plans also restrict participants to eating just 500 calories per day, which alone is both unhealthy and sufficient for rapid weight loss. Health problems that can be caused by following the HGC fad diet include gallstones, edema, and breast swelling in males.

The HCG diet is just one of the more extreme examples of fad diets and why they do not work.

As you probably noticed, some of the diets listed here do include recommendations for healthy food choices. The problem is that, when a diet is designed primarily for weight loss, it is unsustainable for good health. Many, if not most, of the people who use them and do lose weight only gain the weight back again when they return to their normal life and former eating habits.

This is one of the main reasons you should consider intermittent fasting—a lifestyle choice rather than a weight-loss plan.

Chapter 2:

Intermittent Fasting and Women's Health

Everyone who does intermittent fasting talks about it as a lifestyle, not a diet. They come for the weight loss, but stay for the health benefits. —Author unknown

Intermittent fasting is a healthy lifestyle for anyone, but it is especially beneficial for women 50 and older who have gone through menopause and want to stay fit and lose the weight they gained during "The Change."

The Impact of "The Change"

The transition to menopause actually happens in two stages: first perimenopause, when the body prepares to change, and then menopause itself, when menstruation is over. You then enter the period of life called postmenopause.

Perimenopause, menopause, and postmenopause are all a natural part of life, but they represent profound change for a woman, both emotional and physical.

Perimenopause

Perimenopause differs from woman to woman. It normally lasts four years, but for a woman at the extremes it might last for only months or persist for as long as a decade. It can start prematurely for some, as early as the late 30s; for other women, it can start in their 50s.

During perimenopause it is still possible for a woman to get pregnant, but pregnancy becomes less and less likely. This is because your periods become irregular as your ovaries produce less and less estrogen.

A woman's ovaries are the source of the sex hormones estrogen, progesterone, and testosterone. Estrogen and progesterone, the female homes, control menstruation. The body prepares to stop making eggs by producing less and less estrogen.

As a woman's estrogen levels decline, the balance between the hormones estrogen and progesterone gets thrown out of whack. This is the cause of the mood swings that many women experience.

In addition to mood swings and irregular periods, other symptoms of perimenopause include:

- dryness that can affect vaginal health and make sex uncomfortable

- periods that are extra heavy or very light (spotting)

- more frequent urination or leaking

- changes in premenstrual syndrome for women who experience PMS

- hot flashes and night sweats

- insomnia or other sleep problems

- weight gain

There is no cure to stop perimenopause, but there are treatments physicians can offer to provide relief for women who have especially severe symptoms. And, as we will discuss, the IF lifestyle can make a significant difference for you.

Menopause and Postmenopause

You have officially entered menopause when you have not had a period over the course of a full year. For most women, this will be in their 50s.

At this point, you enter the postmenopausal period of your life.

For a period of time after menopause, 75% of women will have hot flashes, either during the day or at night. Hot flashes at night are often called night sweats because they can cause you to perspire so much you wake up in a pool of sweat.

Hot flashes are the result of hormonal changes. During a hot flash, your face may flush, you may sweat, or perhaps feel dizzy or have heart palpitations. Hot flashes after menopause can happen several times a day and you may experience them for as long as a year or two. In extreme cases, they last longer.

After menopause a woman may have a greater risk of cardiovascular disease due to the impact of hormonal changes. Hot flashes can lead to increased blood pressure. Hormonal changes also affect levels of the lipids cholesterol and triglycerides that help repair cells and store energy.

Another result of menopause for many women is osteoporosis, a reduction in bone density that is caused by low levels of calcium in the body. Osteoporosis increases the likelihood of bone fractures.

Weight gain is caused by hormonal changes that affect your metabolism. Your body starts to store more and use less energy. This means that during normal activities you will use fewer calories than you did before, making it harder to burn off the excess energy that your body stores as fat. Typically, most of the weight that is gained settles around your waist (a change that can be compared to the difference between teenage and adult women's bodies).

A possible result of the greater amount of testosterone in that postmenopausal balance of sex hormones is hair loss or thinning on the scalp, combined with an increase in facial hair.

Many women continue to experience vaginal dryness, find sex painful, and have less interest in sex.

There is some thought that menopause also affects memory, but it is not clear if this is due to menopause or is simply a result of aging.

All of these changes, combined with the fact that menopause means the end of possible childbearing—one of the defining characteristics of a young woman—can lead to depression or other mental health problems. But all is not lost! Let's take a look at how IF can help.

The Case for IF

There are prescription and over-the-counter remedies that women can take to alleviate the symptoms of menopause. These include hormone replacement therapies (HRT), sleep aids, vaginal lubricants, and various nutritional supplements.

There are also dietary changes recommended to alleviate symptoms like hot flashes:

- avoiding spicy foods, caffeine, and alcohol

- avoiding smoking and other unhealthy habits

- eating more soybeans, chickpeas, grains, flax, beans, vegetables, and fruits

Let me reiterate, however, that menopause is natural. It is part of the aging process. And in addition to changes related to menopause, your body also experiences a lot of other changes related simply to getting older:

- Your immune system slows down, which means that your body will heal more slowly.

- Your veins and arteries start to stiffen and can become clogged with plaque.

- Even if you do not have osteoporosis, your bones will become less dense and your muscles lose flexibility and strength. This is why many older people get shorter.

- Your digestive system will change. You may have trouble digesting some foods that you used to be able to eat easily (often cheese or spicy food).

- You will experience bladder issues such as leaking or incontinence.

- Memory and cognitive skills decline.

- Your vision and hearing will change, causing you to need glasses (or new glasses) and perhaps to need hearing aids.

- Your teeth and gums get more susceptible to infection and decay.

- Your skin (the largest organ of the body) becomes more fragile and less elastic.

- You are likely to experience changes in sexuality.

- As your metabolism slows, it becomes easier to gain weight.

It is impossible to stop the aging process. But it is possible to take lifestyle steps that will help you stay as healthy as possible and minimize both menopause and aging's effects.

This is where intermittent fasting comes in. We have talked about fasting both as a religious practice and a type of diet. Both are true. Intermittent fasting is a way to incorporate these practices into a healthy lifestyle.

At its core, IF is a discipline that helps you harness the powers of spirituality, good health, and good diet. It is a lifestyle that will ameliorate the effects of menopause and aging so you can be as healthy as possible as long as you can.

Here is just some of the evidence supporting the benefits of IF:

- The website *healthline* cites 10 evidence-based effects of IF (Gunnars, 2016). Among them are:

  o hormonal changes that result in lower insulin and higher human growth hormone (HGH) levels, the stimulation of processes of cellular repair, and the activation of genes

  o weight loss due to increased metabolism and reduced calorie intake

  o lower blood sugar and reduced insulin resistance

  o reduced risk factors for cardiovascular disease

- A study of obese mice that was reported in the journal *Endocrinology* found that a type of IF diet called alternate day fasting (AF) led to significant weight loss and an increase in lean mass (Gotthardt et al., 2016).

- Several studies indicate that IF can result in improved levels of HGH (Mawer, 2019).

- A clinical trial reported in *The American Journal of Clinical Nutrition* found that AF resulted in weight loss, and also improved cardiovascular health with lowered cholesterol, triglyceride levels, and blood pressure levels (Varady et al., 2009).

- In a study involving female mice that was reported in the journal Mechanisms of *Ageing and Development*, the mice that were fed intermittently (4 consecutive days, every 2 weeks) lived about 30% longer than those that were fed daily (Sogawa & Kubo, 2000).

- As reported in *Ageing Research Reviews*, multiple studies show that IF promotes cellular repair functions throughout the body (Bagherniya et al., 2018).

Read on to learn more about the benefits of the IF lifestyle, especially for women 50 and older.

28

Chapter 3:

Fasting Methods

Fasting is the single greatest natural healing therapy. It is nature's ancient, universal 'remedy' for many problems. –Elson Haas, MD

Elson Haas is a physician and a leading proponent of integrative medicine, the branch of medicine that seeks to combine what we know from Western, Eastern, and Natural medical practice—an approach he calls NEW medicine. Dr. Haas is also medical director of the Preventive Medical Center of Marin in California.

Haas recommends intermittent fasting for detoxification, and also as a therapy to treat both medical and life problems. He compares the physical benefits gained from IF to the beneficial effects of taking a vacation.

In the same way that different people are revitalized by different types of vacation, different people will benefit from different types of IF. It is one of the beauties of IF that there is more than one way to practice the discipline. In this chapter, I want to describe eight fasting methods you should know before picking the one that is right for you.

Intermittent fasting (IF) is a term used to describe various plans to control *when* rather than *what* you eat.

To the extent that they include diet recommendations, IF plans often incorporate some elements of the calorie restriction that is the foundation of traditional weight-loss plans. But the goal of IF goes beyond weight loss to incorporate nutritional and physiological goals (I'll discuss these in the next chapter).

Each of the IF plans described below incorporates one of the ideas below for how to define when to eat:

- Time-restricted eating, also called time-restricted feeding: Only eating food during certain hours of the day

- Alternate-day fasting: Consuming no calories at all on fasting days and eating what you want on alternating feast days

- Alternate-day modified fasting: Restricting calories to consume no more than a quarter of your baseline energy need on fasting days, then eating what you want on the alternating days

- Periodic fasting: Fasting one or two days a week and eating what you want on the other days

Keep in mind, the point is not to control calories but to control the hours of the day during which you consume calories. It is true that calories matter. So does your choice of what to eat. But before we talk about healthy diet, let's talk about the various possible IF schedules.

Let me preface this by saying that, especially if you have any pre-existing conditions such as diabetes or cardiovascular disease, be sure to consult a doctor before you decide to adopt an intermittent fasting lifestyle.

12:12

This is a great program for beginners. In addition, working with mice, researchers have found that dieters lost more weight when they followed the 12:12 IF plan (The 12:12 Intermittent Fasting Diet: Can It Really Boost Weight Loss and Flatten Your Tummy?, n.d.).

The 12:12 IF plan follows a schedule that alternates 12 hours of fasting with 12 hours during which you can eat. For example—depending on how much you like eating breakfast or going out to dinner—you might choose to fast between 7:00 p.m. and 7:00 a.m., or you might choose to fast between 10 p.m. and 10 a.m.

This plan is relatively easy to follow because you can arrange your schedule so that the majority of the fasting time occurs when you are asleep. It is also a schedule that can relatively easily accommodate your job, family, and social calendar.

During the fasting period, your body is able to direct resources toward cellular repair, mental clarity, and the consumption of stored energy (fat).

Sometimes your regular schedule will change. You will need to work late or get an early start in the morning. This is where discipline comes in! If you know your schedule will change, you can plan to deal with it. If the change is unexpected, you will need to discipline yourself to stick with the schedule.

You might choose to fit a typical three meals a day into the 12:12 schedule—perhaps breakfast at 8:00 a.m., lunch at 1:00 p.m., and dinner at 7:00 p.m. (that way you will be finished eating by 8:00 p.m.). Or you could choose to eat four or five smaller meals during the same period.

If you look online, you will find many ideas for meal plans that work when you adopt a 12:12 IF schedule.

16:8

This is a popular version of intermittent fasting. Among celebrities who endorse 16:8 IF are Jennifer Aniston, Halle Berry, Hugh Jackman, Vanessa Hudgens, Terry Crews, and Mindy Kaling.

16:8 is a slightly more extreme form of the 12:12 IF program in which practitioners fast for 16 hours and eat within an 8-hour window each day. You can do this every day, once a week, or at whatever interval you prefer.

The trick to succeeding with 16:8 IF is to select an eating window that provides the flexibility you need. For instance, if you are a person who does not like to eat breakfast but would like to be able to go out to dinner, a 12:00 p.m. to 8:00 p.m. or 1:00 p.m. to 9:00 p.m. eating window might work well for you. On the other hand, if breakfast is an important meal for you, consider a 9:00 a.m. to 5:00 p.m. eating window.

One argument for consuming most of the food you eat in the middle of the day is that when you eat at night just before retiring for the day, your body tends to store the calories you eat as fat rather than expending them on daily activity.

Eat Stop Eat

People who follow the Eat Stop Eat IF protocol choose one or two nonconsecutive days each week during which they fast. They eat responsibly during the other five or six days.

5:2 is another name for a 2-day Eat Stop Eat program.

It is possible to plan your Eat Stop Eat schedule so you do not actually have any days where you do not eat at all. For instance, if you choose to fast from 8:00 a.m. on Monday through 8:00 a.m. Tuesday, you can still have an early breakfast on Monday and then eat regular meals on Tuesday.

If you plan to eat foods with high protein and fiber content on Monday morning it will help you postpone hunger pangs on your fasting day. Among the foods that are most filling are meat, fish, oatmeal, eggs, potatoes, and cheese.

It is important to stay hydrated during fast days. Water is the healthiest choice, but people following the Eat Stop Eat plan also drink things like coffee, tea, or zero-calorie soda. Drinking plenty of water is also a way to alleviate hunger because people who are thirsty often think they are feeling hunger pangs.

23/1 (OMAD) Fasting

The 23/1 IF plan is also known as One Meal a Day, or OMAD.

The OMAD diet is just that; you eat one meal each day, and during that one-hour period you can eat whatever you want. Your meal could be breakfast, lunch, or dinner. And you could choose to eat a different meal each day.

This IF diet is relatively extreme and is not recommended for certain people, for instance someone who has diabetes or who takes medication that must be consumed with food more than once a day. Also, OMAD can be a challenging type of IF for someone who is responsible for preparing family meals! But if you are a person who really enjoys going out for meals with friends, or if you eat the kind of protein-rich, nutrient-dense foods that help you feel full for longer periods of time, OMAD might be an IF plan that will work for you.

You can eat whatever you want. Have pizza with the family on pizza and movie night! But in general, eat a balanced diet. Recommended foods for an OMAD meal include lean meat and fish, dark leafy green vegetables, eggs, nuts and seeds, legumes, whole grains, berries, and dark chocolate.

It is a good idea to introduce an OMAD diet slowly. You might start with fasting overnight for 12 hours, then going to 18 hours, and only then graduating to 23/1.

You can also use water or zero-calorie drinks to help with hunger pangs. Keep a mug of coffee and/or bottle of water nearby so that you can drink whenever you want. Some people prefer to use herbal tea. The important thing is to stay hydrated.

2-Day Fast

2-day, or 48-hour, fasting is another of the more extreme methods of IF. In fact, it has the longest fasting time of the IF programs. As the name says, people following the 2-day fast can drink water and zero calorie fluids but do not eat anything for 48 hours.

It is very important to drink plenty of water and other no-calorie fluids, both to help you stay hydrated and avoid hunger pangs.

People following the 2-Day IF plan may want to minimize the waking hours they go without food. One way to do this is to start your fast after a protein-rich dinner on day one so you can sleep, refrain from eating entirely on day two, sleep, and then end your fast with dinner on day three.

A less stringent form of the 2-day fast is called a 2-day Juice Fast. Followers of this plan ingest only fruit or vegetable juices for two days.

After fasting for such a long time, it is also important to start eating again gradually. For example, if you break your fast with dinner on the third day, start with a small appetizer (perhaps some cheese or nuts), and then wait an hour or so before eating a light meal.

Unlike other IF programs with daily or weekly schedules, the 2-Day Fast program is typically followed just once or twice a month.

Because it is such a rigorous, demanding program, be sure to consult a physician before you decide to practice 2-day fasting.

Weekly 24-Hour Fast

People who follow this IF plan choose one day during which they do not eat, but unlike the 2-day fast, they fast every week. There is speculation that this type of fasting mimics the eating pattern of early humans, who ate well after a successful hunt and then fasted until the next meal. The idea is that this pattern of eating is well-suited to our physiology.

The plan is not complicated, but it can be challenging to go an entire day without eating—especially at first.

In order to get the benefits of fasting and still be able to eat something every day, consider scheduling your 24-hour fast starting in the middle of the day. For instance, you could start fasting at noon on Tuesday and fast until noon on Wednesday.

If you are not ready to start 24-hour fasting each week but want to see what the experience is like, look for times that make fasting easier. For some people, fasting is easier and even feels good when they are very full; the day after Thanksgiving might be a good choice. For other people, fasting is easier when their day is busy and they don't have time to think about food.

There is clinical evidence that 24-hour fasting can be therapeutic for patients with Type 2 diabetes. In a small study of three patients at a medical clinic in Canada, the fasting was more extreme and the patients were medically supervised, but the results were dramatic. The patients ate a low-carbohydrate diet, two fasted on alternating days and the third fasted three times a week. On fasting days, they ate only dinner. The other days they ate lunch and dinner. Within a month, all three patients were able to stop taking insulin and became measurably healthier (Furmli et al., 2018).

Meal Skipping

Meal skipping is a form of intermittent fasting that some people do without even knowing it.

Are you a person who skips breakfast because she doesn't like to eat early in the morning? Do you skip lunch because you are so busy at work each day? Surprise. You are intermittent fasting.

If you want to use meal skipping as an IF discipline, how should you choose which meal to skip? Here are some considerations.

Breakfast:

- Skipping this meal extends a fast you started when you went to sleep, and fasting for a longer period of time will earn more benefit in terms of your metabolism.

- This may be an easy meal to skip, especially if your mornings are rushed.

- Most people eat less of their daily calorie intake during breakfast and so may miss breakfast less. And there is evidence that people who skip breakfast do not increase what they eat at lunch and dinner to replace all of the calories saved (Collins, 2020).

- Some athletes recommend not eating before their morning workout to encourage their body to burn more fat (stored energy).

Lunch:

- Skipping lunch can give you the opportunity to experience the metabolic benefits of extending the time between meals twice each day—first from the overnight fast between dinner and breakfast, and then from another fast between breakfast and dinner. I'll go into much more detail about these metabolic benefits in Part 3).

- You will get more benefit from skipping lunch if you do not snack during the day.

Dinner:

- Skipping dinner can be especially difficult because it is ingrained into the social fabric of our lives (dinner with the family, sharing a meal with friends, etc.).

- Dinner tends to be the largest meal of the day, so skipping dinner will potentially save you more calories.

- The body's circadian rhythm is designed for most efficient digestion earlier in the day, meaning that we do not burn calories as efficiently at night, especially when we are at rest.

Warrior Diet

The Warrior Diet was created by Ori Hofmekler, a fitness expert who based the diet on his understanding of nutrition and the idea that ancient warriors did not eat much during the day but then had a big meal at night.

The basic idea is to eat the majority of your calories each day in a four-hour window.

The diet starts in three phases that each lasts one week. Each phase has a list of specific allowed foods.

- Week 1 is detox.

- Week 2 is about adapting to getting fuel from body fat.

- Week 3 is about getting more energy from carbohydrates.

People following the Warrior Diet eat very little during the day, then eat as much as they want from dinner on. However, dieters are supposed to wait 20 minutes after eating dinner to see if they are still hungry before having additional helpings of the same food they had for dinner.

After the first three weeks, dieters can rotate at will among the phase diets.

This is not a highly regarded diet, and it is not advised for certain people, including children, pregnant women or those who are nursing, people who are underweight or have eating disorders, and people with illnesses such as cancer, cardiovascular disease, or diabetes. Interestingly, the Warrior Diet is also not recommended for extreme athletes (Kubala, 2018).

To be successful with any type of intermittent fasting, it is important to choose the protocol that is right for you. You may want to try different IF plans, or switch to a new plan if your life changes.

Next, let's consider what makes IF work.

Part 2:

How IF Works

Chapter 4:

What Happens When We Fast

You are not going to burn body fat if you're eating. –Dr. Jason Fung

Jason Fung is a nephrologist and well-known promoter of intermittent fasting. Beyond endorsing it for overall health, he pioneered the therapeutic use of intermittent fasting combined with a low-carbohydrate diet to treat both diabetes and obesity. As he observed, "Many of today's chronic medical issues are related to diet and obesity, yet treatments are focused on medications and surgeries. If you don't deal with the root cause, the problem never improves. A dietary problem requires a dietary solution" (Jason Fung, MD, n.d.).

Your body always needs energy. Even when you are at rest or asleep, your body is at work, keeping your heart pumping, your lungs taking in oxygen, and all other vital systems going. And yet, we also say that fasting—when you are not providing your body with a new source of energy—is good for you. Fasting is promoted as a way to help you manage your weight, encourage cellular repair, reduce inflammation, boost cognition, and reduce the risk and mitigate symptoms of disease.

To consider why this is, let's examine the five stages of what happens in your body when you fast.

It's a complicated story that experts like physicians and nutritionists study for years to understand. I do not have that expertise. I am simply someone whose life experience has convinced me of the benefits of intermittent fasting. What you will read next is culled from what I have learned from the experts over the years.

The Fed State—Hours 0–4

The fed state is the four hours immediately following a meal. When you are in the fed state, your body is focused on digesting what you ate and absorbing nutrients from it.

You are taking in energy in the form of food, and that food is being digested into proteins, fats, and carbohydrates—the nutrients your body needs.

In order to be absorbed by the body, these essential nutrients must be broken down even further. Proteins become amino acids; they help the body function and build muscles. Fats become fatty acids; they make hormones and cell linings. Carbohydrates become glucose (blood sugar); this is the primary source of energy that powers your cells.

In the fed state, the amount of glucose in your blood goes up.

Nutrients that the body does not need right away are stored against times of scarcity. Fatty acids are stored in fat cells. Unused amino acids can be converted so they can also be stored as fat. Glucose is stored as glycogen in the liver and in fat cells.

Another thing that happens when you are eating is that the pancreas produces insulin. Insulin is a hormone that helps transfer glucose energy into your cells. As you probably know, diabetes is a disease that disrupts how insulin works.

The Early Fasting State—Hours 4–16

The fact that the fed state is triggered whenever you consume food is the reason it is important to consume only water or non-caloric drinks during a fast.

It is also part of the reason that overeating is a problem for people who have diabetes or pre-diabetes, because eating causes the body to overproduce insulin.

But when you do stop eating, after four hours your body moves into a state called early fasting. I have also seen this described as the catabolic state—which is all well and good—but what does it mean?

The catabolic state has to do with metabolism. Your metabolism—the process by which your body uses energy—has two states: anabolic and catabolic. The anabolic state is when the processes of your body are focused on growth. The fed state is anabolic.

The catabolic state is when your body is focused on breaking down nutrients to fuel other activities. During the catabolic state, your body will first use the glycogen (stored glucose) energy that is in your cells. The body then starts to burn energy that is stored as fat.

As the body starts to burn glycogen energy from fat you will notice that you may need to urinate more often. This is because each gram of glycogen is packaged with three grams of water.

At the same time, when you urinate you will excrete electrolytes, which are minerals that conduct electrical signals throughout the body to enable nerve and muscle function and to help regulate the balance of bodily fluids. This is why it is so important to drink plenty of water when you are fasting.

When your body starts to get most of its energy from fat cells instead of blood sugar (glucose), you have entered a state called ketosis. Exactly when ketosis happens depends on the types of food you eat.

For some people, ketosis will start toward the end of the early fasting state. The more fat and protein and less starch and carbs you eat, the sooner ketosis will be triggered.

Achieving a state of ketosis is one of the goals of fasting.

When you are in ketosis, your body creates molecules called ketones or ketone bodies. These ketones are made from fatty acids that replace glucose as a source of fuel. Ketones actually generate more energy with fewer inflammatory by-products than glucose, and this contributes to greater mental clarity and reduced symptoms of such conditions as diabetes and heart disease.

The early fasting state is the one that you will experience during the 12:12 and 16:8 forms of intermittent fasting.

The Fasting State—Hours 16–24

If you have already entered ketosis, the process will accelerate now. If you are not following a moderate, low-carb diet while you are intermittent fasting, you may not enter ketosis until you have fasted for 16–24 hours. But no matter your diet, you will experience ketosis when you enter the fasting state.

During the process of ketosis, you will start to feel less hungry, and this will help you stick with a fasting program.

When you are in ketosis it is also a good time to exercise. During ketosis it is possible to increase the level of ketone in your blood from a concentration of 0.05–0.1 millimoles to as much as 5–7 millimoles. Vigorous cardio exercise such as running will really accelerate the process.

Also, if you fast for a full 24 hours, you will use up your body's store of glycogen. This is desirable because, in addition to burning body fat, your body will also accelerate the process of autophagy.

I mentioned that when certain bodily processes are activated, others are minimized or deactivated. One of the things that happens when you are eating and food is readily available is that the body minimizes the process of autophagy.

The term autophagy comes from two Greek words: *auto* (self) and *phagein* (to eat). The process of autophagy is the process in which the cells clean up by actually eating themselves—breaking down and reusing old, damaged, and abnormal parts.

Autophagy brings a number of health benefits.

You may have heard that the body regenerates itself every seven years. This is because of a process called apoptosis. As the cells in your body get old, they naturally die and are replaced by new cells. Autophagy is an intermediate step. Cells that are damaged or abnormal but too young to die are repaired.

Autophagy breaks down the damaged or abnormal components of cells, repairing them and releasing constituent parts that the body can reuse, such as amino acids, fatty acids, and glucose.

Autophagy also has an anti-inflammatory effect.

I'm sure you are familiar with inflammation from small cuts you have had. It is what happens when your body is injured and the immune system is activated to heal it, and it happens inside as well as outside the body.

Some diseases overstimulate the immune system and cause chronic inflammation. This is a problem for people who suffer from things like rheumatoid arthritis, Type 2 diabetes, cancer, Alzheimer's disease, heart disease, and even asthma. The anti-inflammatory effect of autophagy can provide relief. There is even some thought that it can prevent or help cure cancer.

Because autophagy is stimulated when you reach the fasting state, increased autophagy makes for healthier cells.

This explains how intermittent fasting can actually help you live longer. There has been evidence for this longevity effect in mice since 1945, and now human studies are showing the same effect.

A 2006 study of residents living in elder housing, conducted over three years, compared a control group of people who ate 100% of their recommended calories every day with a test group of people who fasted every other day. On fasting day, they consumed just 56% of their recommended daily calories. The next day, they consumed 144%

of their daily calories. Both groups effectively ate the same amount over the two days but only one group fasted.

The results? There were slightly fewer deaths in the fasting group, but most significantly the people who fasted needed to be hospitalized nearly 45% less often than the control group (Johnson et al., 2006).

Overall reduced autophagy is also one of the changes that happens as we age, so by triggering autophagy, fasting helps reduce the effects of aging. And when fasting is combined with exercise, the effect can be heightened.

Let me emphasize, too, that autophagy happens when your body is burning fat instead of glucose for fuel. This explains how it is possible for intermittent fasters to lose some body fat even if they do not reduce calories or otherwise change their diet.

Entering the Starvation State—Hours 24–72

Prolonged fasting—fasting for more than a day—is extreme and should only be undertaken on the advice and with the supervision of a physician.

That being said, fasting for up to three days does extend the processes of ketosis and autophagy.

Insulin levels continue to be reduced since insulin production is triggered by eating. Too much insulin is associated with insulin resistance and Type 2 diabetes, so lowering insulin levels during a fast can help prevent pre-diabetes and diabetes.

The use of fasting as a treatment for diabetes was pioneered by Dr. Fung, whose quote was at the start of this chapter. Dr. Fung and his colleagues demonstrated the efficacy of fasting in a small study that involved three patients who were being treated for diabetes in a clinic in Canada. The patients followed a program of 24 hour fasting—

actually, 24-hour fasts combined with a low-carb diet. On fasting days, they ate only dinner; on the alternate days they ate dinner and lunch. After less than a month, all 3 patients were able to stop taking insulin and had become measurably healthier (Furmli et al., 2018).

I mentioned that when the brain burns ketones rather than glucose it improves cognitive performance. After 24 hours, that effect is intensified.

Another thing that happens after you have been fasting for 24 hours is that you will have higher levels of human growth hormone (HGH). HGH helps reduce the accumulation of fat, helps the body heal, strengthens your muscles, and improves cardiovascular health.

The combination of autophagy and the increase of HGH is a powerful one because it cleans out old cells while at the same time stimulating the growth of new cells. Since an accumulation of damaged cells is thought to be involved in both Alzheimer's Disease and cancer, it is speculated that this type of fasting can help prevent these diseases. Also, while your body is burning stored fuel instead of glucose, HGH helps preserve lean muscle mass.

It is also known that there is a strong relationship between autophagy and exercise. For example, this is one of the reasons that people who have heart disease are advised to exercise. If you are healthy, studies show that vigorous exercise like bicycling or running a marathon also increases autophagy (Jarreau, 2021).

Starvation—Hours 72+

All of the effects of fasting—lower insulin, ketosis, autophagy, increased HGH—continue after three days of fasting. In fact, your body starts to repair immune cells, revitalizing the immune system. You continue to burn fat, and your mind is clear.

Staying hydrated is critical. And you should not consider this long a fast unless you are healthy and have proper medical supervision.

But starvation is not healthy. In order to keep you alive, your body will start to slow down, which interferes with important metabolic processes.

There are health risks from fasting that lasts for weeks. These include edema, irregular periods, nausea and vomiting, and nutritional deficiencies. But going without eating for three days or more is not really the same as intermittent fasting, and it is not a sustainable lifestyle.

There are many less extreme forms of intermittent fasting which allow you to get the benefits of a fast and do so in a way that you can incorporate into normal daily life.

Let me repeat, I do not advocate starvation. But, by understanding what is happening within your body during each stage of the fasting process, it will be easier for you to stick with an intermittent fasting program. You will understand the many ways you can benefit from it in the long run.

Ending a Fast

If you want to get the maximum benefit from fasting, it is important to pay attention to how to end your fast. The longer the fast, the more important this is because your body needs time to adjust.

If you have fasted for an extended period of time, start with something small like a handful of nuts or some fruit. Then wait about half an hour before eating a full meal.

If you are following one of the more popular forms of IF such as 12:12 or 16:8, break your fast with a well-balanced meal that is high in protein, vegetables, and whole grains, and low on sugar, carbs, and processed food.

The spike in blood sugar you get from carbohydrates will just make you hungry. Do not eat too much, either. After a fast—as always—it is best to eat slowly and drink plenty of water.

Chapter 5:

Understanding the Keys to IF

When you fast good habits gather, like friends who want to help. –Rumi

Rumi was a Persian poet and Sufi Muslim mystic. He celebrated fasting in poetry, as he practiced fasting in life. And his poetry talks of fasting as a source of energy and power.

When I first learned about fasting, I wondered… if fasting is so good for you and the effects of fasting increase the longer you fast, why not recommend maintaining a fast for as long as possible? Why intermittent fasting?

The answer is not just that it is really hard to not eat for a long time. The answer lies in our metabolism and how it works.

Our bodies are made up of trillions of cells that are organized into 78 organs and 10 bodily systems that must all work together (The Live Better Team, 2016). The body coordinates it all through the nervous system to achieve balance (homeostasis), automatically activating certain systems and deactivating others based on what we are doing and what is happening in the environment.

Metabolism is what we call another process: the group of complex biochemical reactions that the body uses to keep us alive and functioning.

As I mentioned earlier, there are two metabolic processes that alternate as we go throughout the day: anabolism (growth) and catabolism (breaking down). When your body heals a wound, that is an anabolic process. When you digest the food you eat, that is a catabolic process.

Intermittent fasting is effective because it takes advantage of these processes.

Two metabolic functions in particular are key to unlocking the benefits of intermittent fasting: the metabolic switch and autophagy. But before I go into detail about how they work, let's get a little background about our body's systems and how they work together.

Systems Working Together

The National Cancer Institute's Surveillance, Epidemiology and End Results (SEER) website has a very helpful overview of the body and its 10 major systems. The systems are:

- Digestive—processes food to be used by the body.

- Cardiovascular—carries blood through the action of the heart and vascular system.

- Respiratory—works with the cardiovascular system to supply oxygen and other gases throughout the body.

- Lymphatic—defends against outside organisms and disease, regulates the balance of fluids, and absorbs fats and fat-soluble vitamins.

- Nervous—transmits electrical signals from the brain to control bodily functions, keeping the body in a state of balance (homeostasis)

- Endocrine—works together with the nervous system, using hormones to send chemical signals to control how the body functions (your metabolism).

- Skeletal—supports and protects the body through a framework of bones, cartilage, tendons, and ligaments.

- Muscular—connects bone, blood vessels, and organs in order to enable movement.

- Urinary—manages the make-up and volume of bodily fluids.

- Reproductive—produces offspring to ensure species survival.

The workings of these systems are an extraordinarily complex, dynamic balance. The balance changes from infancy, through childhood, adolescence, and adulthood. And it changes again for women as we go through menopause.

At all stages, however, we want to do things that will help us to be as healthy as possible. That is where intermittent fasting comes in.

So, with that in mind, let's consider just one of the many series of things that happen when we eat.

Our bodies need energy and we get that energy from food.

All living things are made up of four biological molecules: proteins, carbohydrates, lipids (fats), and nucleic acids. However, different plants and animals put these molecules together in different ways. When we eat, our bodies need to transform the biomolecules we ingested from spinach or eggs into the kinds of proteins, carbs, and fats that make up a human being.

For example, during digestion one of the things that happens is that carbohydrates are turned into glucose. Glucose is transported through the bloodstream to provide energy to the cells. At the same time, the endocrine system signals the pancreas to release the hormone insulin, which is needed in order to transfer glucose from the blood into the cells.

If the body does not need any more energy, insulin triggers the liver to store the unneeded glucose as glycogen.

Then, when our bodies need energy but there is not a lot of glucose in our blood, our pancreas releases the hormone glucagon, which triggers glycogen molecules in the liver to release glucose. It also signals the body to create glucose from amino acids, and prevents your liver from creating more glycogen. And, if needed to keep things in balance, the pancreas will release insulin.

Our bodies are able to both use food as we are eating it and store extra nutrients away for when food is scarce. This is a system that evolved as a survival mechanism.

In the wild, looking for food takes time and energy. Wolves feast when food is available and fast until the next meal. Bears gorge all summer and live on what their bodies stored as fat when they hibernate in the winter. Similarly, prehistoric humans experienced times of feast or famine, and our bodies are built for that.

Human biology is based on what we call the circadian rhythm—the body's 24-hour clock that helps regulate our metabolism. Sleeping and fasting recharge our system. So, if you eat your last meal of the day at 7:00 p.m. and do not eat again until 7:00 a.m., fasting is a normal part of your day.

The problem is, many people eat three meals and also snack all day and into the night. Even if you are just grazing—eating a little bit every time—this eating pattern means that your body will never fall into a state of fasting.

That is why intermittent fasting is so beneficial. By leveraging the processes of the metabolic switch and autophagy, IF helps restore your body's natural rhythms.

The Metabolic Switch

The metabolic switch refers to what happens when your body switches into ketosis, which as you know, means that you are getting your energy directly from glucose stored as fat instead of from glucose in your blood. On average, this happens 12 hours after you start to fast.

Energy fuels everything that you do, and your body naturally uses the food source most readily available. When you eat, that is glucose, which is water soluble and easily transported. There is nothing wrong with this. We need to ingest fuel and experience the anabolic, or growth, state.

Growing babies and children need to eat all the time. As adults we do not have the same nutritional needs, but growth is still important for us. It is how we build up our strength and how the body heals a broken bone or a paper cut.

Problems arise, however, when glucose becomes our only source of energy. When this happens, our bodies get out of balance, which can lead to obesity and other disease.

You can address the problem of being overweight with a calorie-restricted (CR) diet, and calorie restriction does lead to weight loss and has other health benefits. However, it can be really tough to stay on a CR diet. This is why dieters using CR plans so often gain the weight back when they return to their normal routines.

There is also a growing body of evidence that calorie restriction alone cannot provide the same systemic benefits as intermittent fasting, in large part because of the metabolic switch. The research shows that, in addition to promoting weight loss and improving metabolism, IF can provide health benefits such as (Anton et al., 2018).:

- reduced risk of cardiovascular problems due to reduced cholesterol and triglycerides (lipids) in the blood

- reduced inflammation blood clotting in your veins (thrombophlebitis)

- reduced inflammation from osteoarthritis,

- promote the healing of serious skin wounds (refractory dermal ulcers),

- fewer adverse reactions during elective surgery, and

- preservation of lean muscle mass during weight loss

A number of serious negative side effects are also reported in the literature, but only when associated with extreme fasting over a matter of weeks, not with intermittent fasting.

Think back to our prehistoric ancestors. When food was scarce, they needed extra energy and mental clarity in order to hunt successfully. If being hungry had made them weak and lethargic, they would have been in trouble. When they were hungry was when they needed to be at their best. And when they were hungry, they were fueling their bodies from stored fat.

This explains why people who fast report feeling energized and mentally alert. Their bodies are getting the fuel they need. And their brains are being fueled by an energy source that is more efficient than glucose.

What does that mean? It means that you are getting your energy from ketones made from fatty acids stored in your liver. Ketones provide more energy and cause less inflammation.

Ketones used by the body as fuel also increase something called brain derived neurotrophic factor (BDNF). BDNF is a molecule that helps regulate how the brain uses energy and is also involved with memory and learning. Decreased BDNF is associated with things like Alzheimer's and Parkinson's disease. Increased BDNF is associated with improved cognitive function.

The brain actually uses most of our energy, so having a more efficient energy source can promote overall physical performance as well.

Flipping the metabolic switch is good for you.

Autophagy

And this brings us to the second key to the benefits of intermittent fasting: autophagy.

We know that insulin, the "master hormone of the fed state," inhibits autophagy (Rabinowitz & White, 2010). But as Robert Skinner explains, autophagy ramps up when you fast.

Robert Skinner is a researcher and sports scientist who wrote the book *The If Diet*. He explains it like this:

> "Intermittent fasting definitely and massively increases autophagy. And thanks to our caveman history, it thrived. In times of little food, lysosomes would race around the body looking for damaged cells, pre-diseased cells, and cells which weren't doing much. It would chop them apart – into their smallest parts – and either burn them for energy, or use them to repair other areas. Simply, it would perform miracles without any outside help." (Geurin, 2021)

Lysosomes are fundamental to autophagy because they are the parts of the cell that are able to break down, digest, and remove waste.

Autophagy is the body's self-cleaning process. It happens in the background all the time.

Autophagy is also a process that is robust when you are young. But it starts to decrease as you age, so being able to stimulate the process has anti-aging benefits that will help you stay healthy longer.

Cleaning up cells and keeping them healthy is an important biological task. It helps to prevent cancer, rheumatoid arthritis and other autoimmune diseases, Parkinson's and other neurodegenerative diseases, diabetes, and strokes and other cardiovascular diseases.

Too much autophagy (like too much of pretty much anything) can be bad for you, for instance, by causing cells to grow abnormally. However, promoting a healthy amount of autophagy is important, especially as we age.

I talked earlier about the cells in your body dying and being replaced every seven years. This is a broad generalization and not entirely true. Different cells live different amounts of time. There are cells, like some in your blood, stomach, or skin, that regenerate in a matter of days or weeks. Others last for years.

Still others, like some in your heart, brain, and eyes, are designed to last for your lifetime. Autophagy is critical for keeping these cells healthy!

Both calorie-restricted diets and intermittent fasting can stimulate autophagy. The problem is that healthy people following a CR diet will need to cut from 10% to as much as 40% of the calories they eat each day in order to induce autophagy. This can be difficult to sustain.

On the other hand, if you follow an IF lifestyle with time-restricted eating, there are programs in which you will go for 12, or even 24, hours without food. This will allow you to stimulate autophagy and still eat at least one meal each day.

In fact, a study conducted at Columbia University and reported in the journal *Nature*, demonstrated that, depending on the fasting schedule, IF increased autophagy and actually improved the health and extended the life of fruit flies by 13% for males and 18% for females (Mayer, 2021).

Fruit flies were used because they have a similar circadian rhythm to ours (awake in the day, asleep at night), they have about 70% of the same genes related to disease, and they only live for two months so it is easier to study their lifespan.

What the researchers discovered was that one particular kind of intermittent fasting extended lifespan and that was a program where the flies alternated between fasting for 20 hours on one day, and eating as they wanted for 24 hours the next day. But... this only worked if the flies fasted all night and did not start eating again until lunch the next day.

There were no benefits to flies that fasted during the day but ate at night, flies that only had access to food for 12 hours during the day, or flies that alternated 24 hours of fasting with 24 hours of feeding.

Autophagy was not increased unless the flies fasted at night. This certainly supports the idea that sleep recharges you! And it clearly indicates the likelihood that a similar IF program will have similar benefits for humans.

Also, as we will discuss later, there are things you can do such as diet and exercise that will make autophagy ramp up sooner rather than later when you are intermittent fasting.

The bottom line is, if you want to get the best results from intermittent fasting, you need to make that metabolic switch and try to reach autophagy when you can.

Part 3:

Benefits of IF

Chapter 6:

Weight Loss

Fasting is like spring cleaning for your body. —Jentezen Franklin

I think Franklin's analogy makes sense because, like spring cleaning, intermittent fasting clears out things that are old and damaged or that you no longer need. One of these things is excess weight.

I have been emphasizing many of the other benefits to be gained from intermittent fasting, but weight loss was certainly a major plus for me. And I know that weight loss is an issue for many women when we are over 50. So, let's consider how and why you can lose weight with intermittent fasting.

Reduced Caloric Intake

When you are intermittent fasting—even if you do not change anything else about your diet—you are likely to lose weight. Simply limiting when you eat will help you drop extra pounds because you are not eating so often.

Many people whose goal is weight loss choose to follow calorie restricted diets. These are diets that limit how many calories you eat and also require you to eat foods that provide adequate nutrition.

In the previous chapter I mentioned that calorie-restricted diets have many of the same benefits you get from IF. A National Institute of Aging (NIA) review of research findings summarized the benefits of a calorie-restricted diet, if it is adopted as a lifestyle (Calorie Restriction and Fasting Diets: What Do We Know?, 2018).

- If you stick with the diet, you will lose weight.

- Experiments with animals—from worms and flies to mice and monkeys—have shown that a CR diet can delay and reduce effects of-aging, and even increase life span.

- The major study of human subjects following a CR diet was the Comprehensive Assessment of Long-term Effects of Reducing Intake of Energy (CALERIE) clinical trial sponsored by NIA. Participants were asked to restrict calories by 25%, but in practice they were only able to maintain a 12% calorie reduction. However, they were able to stay on the diet for two years. The results?

  - At the end of the study, and in a follow-up two years later, participants had lost about 10% of their starting weight and most were able to keep it off.

  - Participants had lower risk of disease as evidenced by reduced cholesterol levels and blood pressure.

  - There were some adverse effects such as reductions in bone density, ability to maximize the body's use of oxygen (aerobic capacity), and lean body mass. But we know that these effects of weight loss can be countered with exercise.

  - Participants also reported improved sleep, mood, sexuality, and overall satisfaction with life.

We are also learning about the mechanisms in the body that are responsible for the health benefits of a CR diet. Among the processes known to be affected are:

- how the body metabolizes sugar for fuel

- how the immune system uses inflammation, the process intended to deal with invasion from bacteria and viruses

- how the body keeps proteins healthy

- how the body turns genes on and off to make specialized cells and help cells react to the environment

- how the body metabolizes, or uses, oxygen

The basis of calorie restriction is simple arithmetic: the less energy in (fewer calories you eat), the more energy out (more stored calories you will use).

Our bodies need energy to function. We get that energy from food in the form of three nutrients: proteins, carbohydrates, and fats. The amount of energy we eat and use is measured in calories.

When we eat, some of the nutrients are used right away. And as you know, what is not used, the body stores as fat. If you want to lose weight, you need to use more calories than you eat. The rule of thumb is to cut 500 calories a day in order to lose half a pound to one pound a week. However, this will vary based on your age, body type, gender, and activity level.

With intermittent fasting, the goal is for your body to make up the difference between calories eaten and calories needed by using up some fat. One of the issues with losing weight simply by counting calories is that you lose a combination of fat, water weight, and lean muscle. And as your weight decreases, you may need to cut more calories in order to keep losing.

The three things you can do to cut calories are to:

1. eat smaller portions.

2. avoid food that is high in calories but low in nutrition (like sodas or chips).

3. replace a high-calorie food choice (like waffles) with a lower calorie choice (like eggs).

However, when you count calories, it is possible to reduce calories without having to give up every food indulgence you enjoy. And if you increase how much you exercise along with cutting calories, you will lose even more.

Reduced Hunger

When I started intermittent fasting, I was really worried about being hungry all the time. What I learned is that there are things you can do to manage feelings of hunger. And the more I stayed with the program, the less hungry I felt.

The truth is, I do not think I had ever really been hungry. I always had three meals a day unless I was very busy or for some other reason chose to miss a meal. But my body was conditioned to expect a meal.

That conditioning was appetite, not hunger. I saw an interesting blog about this that explains appetite vs hunger in terms of Pavlov and how he was able to condition dogs to salivate when he rang a bell (Lett, 2021). This is what happens to us if we eat three meals a day at around the same time every day. Our bodies become conditioned to expect food, and we think we are hungry.

At other times we might tell ourselves that we are hungry when what we are is stressed, emotional, or bored.

Our bodies have a hormone called ghrelin that tells our brain that our stomach needs food, which makes us feel hungry. There is also a hormone called leptin that tells our brain that we are full. These hormones work together to help maintain our bodies' balance of energy.

This hormonal balance will be affected when you start intermittent fasting. But your body will adjust to your new eating pattern, and you will no longer feel so hungry during a fast.

There are also things you can do to control the very real hunger pangs that intermittent fasting will induce. After all, the goal is to make yourself hungry so your body will start burning stored fat.

Luckily, real hunger pangs only last for a while—usually 20 minutes or less.

Here are some things you can do to minimize your hunger.

- Eat a diet that is low in carbohydrates and high in fat and includes moderate amounts of protein. This is the basis of a healthy diet that will make you feel full, and help keep your blood sugar levels in balance. Think about it. Don't you feel more replete after a breakfast of eggs and whole wheat toast than you do after a breakfast of donuts or sugared cereal?

- Reduce stress. Sleep deprivation causes stress, so get plenty of sleep. Stress can make you feel hungry because your body is preparing to deal with a threat and sends out signals that you need fuel.

- Hydrate. Sometimes you think you are hungry when, in fact, you are thirsty. Make sure to drink plenty of water before you start a fast, and keep plenty of liquids at hand. Drinking will make your stomach full, which alleviates hunger. But be sure not to drink too much. Drinking more than three quarts of water a day will flush electrolytes that your body needs to function properly.

- In addition to water, you might drink coffee or tea. Another thing you might try while you are adjusting to the experience of fasting is something called "bulletproof coffee." This is a high-fat coffee drink that was popularized along with the keto/low

Carb diet. And the fats in the coffee will not inhibit ketosis or autophagy.

- If you do get over-hydrated and lose electrolytes, try putting a little bit of salt on your tongue. Then the next time you fast, be sure to put plenty of salt on your pre-fasting meal. You might drink some bone broth. And you can consider taking a magnesium and potassium supplement before and while you fast.

- Limit how much alcohol you drink the day before a fast. Alcohol can mess with your hormones and blood sugar, with the effect that it makes you feel hungry. It has plenty of calories, but little nutritional value, because it prevents nutrients from being fully absorbed.

- Stay busy. Have you ever had the experience of being so involved with what you are doing that you simply forgot to eat? Staying busy will distract you from feeling hungry. So, make a plan to fill your time on fasting days.

Over time, you will find that hunger is less and less of an issue.

Repaired Metabolism

Research shows that both prolonged fasting and calorie-restricted diets have been shown to slow down your metabolism. Studies of participants in the TV show *The Biggest Loser* found that, while people lost a lot of weight on CR diets, they regained most, if not all of the weight lost. They also experienced a lasting drop in metabolism. But intermittent fasting can actually increase metabolism (West, 2021).

I think this relates to what we were talking about earlier: the evolutionary basis for fasting in the dietary patterns of early humans.

Metabolism is the process of converting nutrients into energy. Intermittent fasting does not slow your metabolism. Rather, it changes your body's source of energy. In fact, in a study done at the University of Vienna participants who followed a three-day intermittent fast actually increased their metabolism by 14% (Trumpfeller, 2020).

We also know that intermittent fasting increases levels of human growth hormone (HGH). HGH signals the body to break down lipids and other fatty acids to be used as fuel (Horne et al., 2015).

Increased Autophagy

I will not repeat the discussion of autophagy from the previous chapter, but let me just emphasize that your body stores fat in order to use it, and autophagy is one of the body's processes to do just that.

Autophagy triggers the release of glucagon, and as you may recall, that is the hormone that tells the liver to retrieve glucose stored in glycogen.

Repaired Insulin Resistance

In Chapter 4, I talked about Dr. Jason Fung and his use of intermittent fasting to successfully treat diabetes. Dr. Fung pioneered this therapeutic approach and is a big proponent of intermittent fasting.

Diabetes is a disease that interferes with how your body uses energy because it affects your ability to respond to insulin, the hormone that tells your cells that there is glucose in the blood ready to be used.

Insulin resistance is a condition in which your cells don't get the message. The level of glucose in your blood rises, and that triggers your body to store unneeded glucose as fat.

Unfortunately, being overweight can trigger insulin resistance. By helping you lose weight, intermittent fasting can help repair problems with insulin resistance.

Overall Findings

A review published by Harvard's T. H. Chan School of Public Health found that calorie restriction and intermittent fasting did both promote weight loss (Diet Review: Intermittent Fasting for Weight Loss, 2018).

The problem with calorie restriction is two-fold. First, people who succeed in losing weight often regain the weight when they transition from a dieting lifestyle to their normal daily life. Second, when people stay on a very low-calorie diet for a long period of time, their metabolism adapts to the new diet and, if they need to lose more weight, they need to restrict calories even further.

There is no magic number to tell you how much weight you will lose with intermittent fasting, and most people who start IF do not do so with a specific weight-loss goal in mind. Intermittent fasting is much more a lifestyle choice than a weight loss program.

However, when you do incorporate intermittent fasting into your life you will most likely lose weight.

Many IF regimens incorporate guidelines for a healthy diet that, in itself, promotes shedding excess pounds. We know that (depending on your starting weight) weight loss of one or two pounds a week is the healthiest. Research shows that people who adopt intermittent fasting achieve this kind of slow, steady weight loss that lasts—typically losing about a pound a week over ten weeks (Trumpfeller, 2020).

Intermittent fasting focuses on losing fat rather than losing weight. This matters because when weight loss is achieved solely through calorie restriction, dieters will lose weight from water, muscle, and organ tissue as well as fat—especially when their goal is rapid weight loss.

The key to weight loss with intermittent fasting is to combine fasting with a healthy diet and exercise. This way you will burn excess fat and maintain lean muscle mass.

Chapter 7:

Brain and Mental Health

Fasting is a calming experience. It is restful…relieves anxiety and tension. It is rarely depressing and it is often downright exhilarating. –Allan Cott, M.D.

Psychiatrist Allan Cott was a pioneer in the field of orthomolecular psychiatry, a type of alternative medicine that relies on nutritional supplements. He also introduced the Russian fasting treatment in the United States, and used it to successfully treat mentally ill patients suffering from manic depression.

This quote from Dr. Cott captures one of the most amazing things that I learned when I discovered intermittent fasting: the powerful restorative effect IF has on our brain and mind.

I was surprised to discover for myself that, when I fasted, I actually felt mentally sharper. Then I talked to folks who told me similar stories. One friend, for instance, said that when she had a presentation to make or a particularly important morning at work, instead of eating a big breakfast she would just have a cup of coffee and wait to eat until her work was done.

In this chapter I am going to explore the research into how and why intermittent fasting has these kinds of effects on the brain.

Brain Health

I have already discussed how, when you are in a state of ketosis, your brain is energized by getting energy from ketones. I talked about the likely evolutionary basis for our being able to achieve peak performance when we were forced to fast through lack of food.

As you know, after about 12 hours IF triggers a state of ketosis, during which the body derives energy from stored fat rather than blood glucose. The ketones that are created as an energy source are particularly healthy for the brain.

Improvements in Overall Brain Function

An article on the website of Radboud University in the Netherlands lists several other aspects of intermittent fasting that also help the brain (Klimars, 2019):

- About six hours after starting a fast, the body releases an increased level of human growth hormone (HGH). This matters because, when the body's store of glucose is low, proteins as well as fats can be used to create ketone. HGH affects the metabolism to encourage the body to burn fat rather than protein.

- HGH also encourages the body toward autophagy, which as we discussed is very important for long-lived neurons in the brain.

- Intermittent fasting increases BDNF in the brain, which improves cognitive function.

A literature review in the journal *Nutrients* summarized research into the benefits of IF in the treatment and cure of diseases related to the brain. It cites human clinical trials in which IF reduced symptoms and progression of multiple sclerosis, Alzheimer's disease, and epilepsy. It also discusses promising animal research that indicates IF can benefit mental conditions such as autism spectrum disorder (ASD), anxiety, and emotional disorders (Gudden et al., 2021).

To summarize the mechanisms that IF stimulates in the brain, while the brain is using ketones for fuel, signals are sent that increase the rate of BDNF production. When BDNF is increased several things happen:

- Neurons are stimulated to make new connections (facilitating learning and memory).

- Something called mitochondrial biogenesis is increased, which means that new mitochondria are produced. Mitochondria are the parts of the cell that create the chemical energy used to fuel the cell's functioning.

- Cellular stress resistance is increased. This means that cells are better able to react to damage from the environment, including through autophagy.

- Chemical changes curb the growth of cells and proteins, another stimulus to repair cells through autophagy.

- Improved sensitivity to insulin (which helps cells use blood sugar) helps neurons in the brain use glucose more effectively. This is a benefit for diabetics, and for older people, for whom insulin sensitivity decreases with age.

Homeostasis and metabolic balance in the body are tied to our natural circadian rhythms, triggered by the cycle of night and day. In the modern world, these rhythms are disturbed by extended hours of eating, 24-hour lighting, and shifting patterns of work. The exact mechanisms are difficult to understand without advanced knowledge of physiology, but during fasting, our bodies are able to re-regulate insulin secretion and the balance of anabolic and catabolic processes (growth and breaking down).

We are learning a lot about the importance of the gut microbiome— the world of microorganisms that live in our digestive tract. This microbiome is important to insulin sensitivity, immune responses, and brain health. The health of the microbiome depends on a circadian clock that is affected by when we eat. For example, eating too close to sleep (our recharge time), reduces the diversity of the microbiome, which makes it less effective. Intermittent fasting has been shown to improve the health of the microbiome, and so contribute to improved brain health.

Protection Against Disease

In addition to its benefits for people who are healthy, intermittent fasting can ameliorate the impact or perhaps even prevent the development of diseases that affect the brain.

IF can ameliorate neurodegenerative diseases:

- We do not know exactly how Alzheimer's disease works, but we do know that it involves the build-up of plaques and protein in the brain and progressive decline of mental abilities. We do not know how, but there is evidence that intermittent fasting improves symptoms by suppressing inflammation and increasing the use of energy from ketones.

- Multiple sclerosis (MS) causes reduced executive functioning, attention, information processing, and long-term memory. We know that it affects more people in the West, and that it is likely associated with nutrient deficiencies. Research shows that IF was able to actually reverse the progression of MS, in experiments with mice and in human trials. It is speculated that this is due to improvements in the gut microbiome.

- Parkinson's disease affects both motor control and brain function, and symptoms are aggravated by inflammatory reactions in the body and brain. One of the results of Parkinson's is a decrease in dopamine, which transmits chemical messages between your body and brain. Intermittent fasting may help alleviate symptoms through the increase in BDNF, which has been shown to improve dopamine levels.

IF is therapeutic for people with injuries involving the central nervous system:

- Ischemic stroke is the most common kind of stroke. It stops oxygen to the brain, and brain cells die—nearly two million every minute—which can lead to impaired brain function. In experiments with rodents, those who had been on an IF diet for three months had less cognitive loss after a stroke than did mice eating at will. The ketones in the brain also reduce inflammation. Inflammation causes swelling that can exacerbate the effects of the stroke. Reduced inflammation resulted in better outcomes.

- Autism spectrum disorder (ASD) inhibits language, communication, and emotional regulation. Children with ASD also often have gastrointestinal problems as well. Based on the relationship between IF and the gut microbiome, research is being done to investigate the ability of IF to mitigate symptoms of ASD.

- Epilepsy is a disorder that causes seizures, during which patients lose muscle control and may also lose consciousness. There is growing evidence from animal studies that IF reduces the incidence and impact of seizures by improving metabolism and inflammation in the brain.

In sum, intermittent fasting is good for brain health.

Studies of people fasting during Ramadan reported less depression, stress, and anxiety. A study of people 60+ with mild cognitive impairment (MCI) found that people who followed IF over three years no longer had MCI symptoms (Smart, 2022).

We do not yet know exactly how it works, but is that a reason not to experience the benefits for yourself?

Mental Health

I am making a distinction here between brain health and mental health. These terms are often used interchangeably, but for my purposes I am talking about how the brain works (brain health) and how the brain expresses cognition and emotion (mental health).

In addition to its impact on brain health, intermittent fasting is also associated with improved mental health and psychological well-being.

Improved Mood

As you know if you have gone or are going through "the change," menopause can be an emotional roller-coaster.

Perhaps you have felt irritable, sad, tense, or anxious. You may have a hard time concentrating, feel tired, lack motivation, or bounce between moods.

Mood and anxiety disorder is an umbrella term for a wide range of conditions that affect mental health. By increasing levels of BDNF (which facilitates communication in the brain), intermittent fasting can improve your mood.

How does it work?

You may have heard of serotonin, a chemical that acts as a mood stabilizer. It can help you feel good. A lot of the medicine that is used to treat mood disorders includes serotonin. People take serotonin supplements to help improve mood and sleep.

Serotonin and BDNF work together to strengthen brain activity. They also affect mood. When BDNF and serotonin cannot communicate effectively, BDNF encourages the survival of serotonin, which helps you feel more calm, happy, and emotionally stable.

After several days, intermittent fasting also leads to higher levels of endorphins. Endorphins are hormones related to fitness and pain relief (think runner's high). They elevate your mood, especially after cardio exercise.

Reduced Anxiety and Stress

Stress is an important human response. It is nature's way to alert you to danger, triggering an automatic reaction we call fight or flight. But the stress reaction is being disrupted in the modern world.

For our prehistoric ancestors, stress was triggered by life-threatening physical threats. We reacted to the danger and the stress went away. Today, however, most threats we face are not immediately life-threatening. And all too often these threats persist. This can lead to an unhealthy state of chronic stress, with the result that stress and anxiety are among the most prevalent disorders affecting quality of life for people today.

There is growing evidence that intermittent fasting has a positive effect to reduce anxiety and stress. For example, in studies of people who observe Ramadan, fasting was reported to have a positive effect to reduce stress (Berthelot et al., 2021).

It is believed that IF relieves anxiety and stress by supporting the health of our gut microbiome. Fasting also increases your levels of BDNF. This increases the plasticity in your brain, and this makes it easier to adjust your mood.

Reduced Depression

Intermittent fasting has been shown to help reduce depression and, again, BDNF is a factor.

BDNF is what is called a transducer, something that converts energy from one form to another. In terms of technology, a microphone or a thermometer is a transducer. In terms of biology, a transducer is a receptor that converts a signal between the inside and outside of a cell.

A study reported in the journal Neuropharmacology found that BDNF acts as a transducer to facilitate the efficacy of antidepressant drugs (Björkholm & Monteggia, 2016).

This makes sense because research indicates that one cause of depression is a lack of what is called adaptive plasticity in the brain—that is, a reduced ability to respond to changes in the environment (Dwivedi, 2009).

BDNF plays a major role in neuroplasticity, and intermittent fasting is known to increase BDNF levels in the brain. Neuroplasticity is the ability of the brain to make new connections, which is how we learn and how the brain can recover from injury.

Even without drugs, IF can have an anti-depressive effect.

In sum, intermittent fasting is beneficial to your brain in many ways—from improving your mood to delaying cognitive decline.

Chapter 8:

Protection From Infection and

Illness

He who eats until he is sick must fast until he is well. –English Proverb

A proverb is a short, memorable statement of common wisdom, passed down over time. There is no author. They are not always stated in the same way. They are not meant to be literal. They are meant, rather, to express ideas that connect to something with deep roots in our experience.

Fasting for good health is one of those ideas.

The point is not to starve yourself when you do not feel well. It is to take advantage of your body's own process for healing and renewal.

For example, the proverb says to "fast until he is well," but what we know today is that intermittent, or short-term fasting puts cells under a mild form of stress that is beneficial because it triggers your body to release energy that has been stored as fat. Then when you stop fasting, your body has time to recover from that stress (Griffith, 2017).

In this chapter I would like to take a look at research behind four examples of how these benefits of intermittent fasting provide protection from infection and illness.

Covid-19

I cannot write this today without talking about the health challenge of our decade—Covid-19.

In the United States alone, more than 94 million cases have been reported, and more than a million of these people died (The New York Times, 2022). Still others, estimated currently in the tens of millions, contracted long-haul Covid and are living with chronic aftereffects (Long-Haul COVID Deserves More Attention, UTSW Expert Says, 2022).

At the same time, I saw a study reported in the journal *Pharmacy Times* that found that people who regularly practice intermittent fasting and contracted Covid had much better outcomes (Mulrooney, 2022).

Data were collected prior to the availability of vaccines from a healthcare registry for a system of hospitals in Utah. Many of the system's patients had practiced fasting regularly for decades as part of their Mormon faith (Intermountain Healthcare, 2022).

205 of the patients in the registry contracted Covid. 73 of these reported that they fasted on the first Sunday of every month, following a form of 2-day fasting. Fasters eat no food and drink only water for 48 hours.

The patients who fasted were not protected from contracting Covid, but their cases were less severe as measured by a noticeably lower rate of hospitalization.

How does Covid work to mitigate the severity of Covid? Dr. Horne, Director of Cardiovascular and Genetic Epidemiology at the hospital, identified three mechanisms at work:

- The first is autophagy. Fasting routinely gives a boost to the body's self-cleaning process.

- Second is the anti-inflammatory effect of fasting, which protects against the extreme inflammation that is caused by Covid.

- And third is ketosis. Linoleic acid is a fatty acid that is a source of ketone. As Dr. Horne explains it, "There's a pocket on the surface of SARS-CoV-2 that linoleic acid fits into – and can make the virus less able to attach to other cells" (Intermountain Healthcare, 2022). SARS-C0V-2 is the virus that causes Covid.

Other researchers who were looking for potential ways to combat Covid reviewed existing evidence of the benefits of IF to determine the likelihood that intermittent fasting would effectively protect against Covid. They reported that the mechanisms of autophagy and increased immune response both have great promise (Hannan et al., 2020).

This is why, leading into the month of Ramadan, the website of the Cleveland Clinic in Abu Dhabi reassured their Muslim readers that fasting has a protective effect against Covid (Cleveland Clinic Staff, 2021b).

We also know that people with preexisting conditions such as cancer, diabetes, and hypertension are more vulnerable to Covid. Just as intermittent fasting protects against and mitigates the effects of these diseases, it can provide similar protection against Covid.

The Immune System Connection

There is a strong connection between fasting and the immune system.

We know that one benefit of intermittent fasting is that it strengthens the immune system, and one reason for this has to do with something called immunosenescence. Immunosenescence means that the immune system deteriorates as we age. For people 65 and older, this deterioration often means the onset of chronic, low-grade inflammation.

Research shows that intermittent fasting can reduce the impact of immunosenescence by reducing inflammation and improving the ability of the immune system to respond to injury and disease (Longo & Cortellino, 2020).

Let's consider how and why.

Fasting Regenerates Immune Cells

During autophagy, defective cells are recycled. Among these are any defective white blood cells.

Unlike red blood cells that carry oxygen throughout the body, white blood cells are part of the immune system. Their purpose is to fight infection.

Since our body needs a healthy level of white blood cells, the destruction of damaged ones then triggers the generation of new, healthy white blood cells. This regeneration of our white blood cells boosts immunity.

Fasting Reduces Inflammation

Autophagy reduces inflammation because the damaged cells that are digested are one cause of inflammation.

A quick online search will return many examples of studies that show the ability of intermittent fasting to reduce inflammation:

- Researchers at Mount Sinai in New York have studied the mechanism by which intermittent fasting reduces inflammation, both improving chronic inflammatory diseases and maintaining the immune system's ability to respond as needed. (Mount Sinai Researchers Discover That Fasting Reduces Inflammation and Improves Chronic Inflammatory Diseases, 2019). Intermittent fasting was shown to reduce the number of specialized immune cells called monocytes that increase inflammation. It was also shown to trigger monocytes to power down, making them less inflammatory.

- A study that followed Muslims during the month of Ramadan found that intermittent fasting decreased inflammation. Both men and women who fasted had more HDL, the "good" cholesterol that helps remove too much other cholesterol from the blood. They also had significantly lower levels of homocysteine, a known marker for inflammation (Yılmaz & Kayançiçek, 2018).

- In another study of patients who suffered from obesity and asthma, an alternate-day intermittent fasting regimen was shown to significantly reduce markers of inflammation. This improvement was measured after only two weeks and continued for the eight weeks of the study (Johnson et al., 2007).

Fasting Helps Reduce Chronic Pain

A literature review of research on intermittent fasting revealed how IF can be a non-pharmacological, non-invasive regimen to help reduce chronic pain (Caron et al., 2022).

The researchers noted that chronic pain is associated with many diseases known to be ameliorated by intermittent fasting (arthritis, cancer, diabetes, etc.). There are six different types of pain:

1. mechanical (damaged cartilage between joints, muscle strain, broken bones)

2. inflammatory (fluid build-up, damaged or swollen tissue)

3. visceral (pain in the internal organs such as menstrual pain)

4. ischemic (caused by a lack of blood to some part of the body)

5. neuropathic (injured nervous tissue)

6. centralized (caused by malfunction of pain signaling in the nervous system)

And intermittent fasting was shown to reduce all six types of pain.

Mechanical pain is relieved in two ways: weight loss and insulin reduction. Weight loss reduces pressure on affected joints. Insulin is known to be involved in the deterioration of cartilage, so insulin reduction helps preserve cartilage.

Inflammatory pain is ameliorated by IF's known anti-inflammatory effect.

IF's role in strengthening the gut microbiome can help with visceral pain.

Ischemic pain can be improved by IF's anti-inflammatory effect.

One way neuropathic pain is relieved is by the improvement in neuroplasticity that results from increased levels of BDNF. Specifically, synaptic neuroplasticity can help your body adjust to better handle pain.

Centralized pain can be alleviated by an increase in levels of serotonin and endorphins, the same chemical messengers that contribute to improved mood; and also, by the fact that with less pain, patients can get a better night's sleep.

Effects on Cancer and Cancer Treatment

Intermittent fasting has been shown to reduce the risk of cancer and also reduce the side effects of cancer treatments.

Reduced Cancer Risk

Both calorie-restricted diets and intermittent fasting can help to reduce the risk of developing cancer. A literature review conducted at the University of California San Francisco explains why IF is a better therapeutic choice (Cancer and Fasting, 2014).

Dr. Valter Longo is a gerontologist and researcher at the University of Southern California who studies cancer and other diseases related to aging. He found that CR without malnutrition is a particularly powerful way that diet can be used to protect against cancer. However, CR diets do not produce cancer-fighting benefits quickly. And in addition, they are not healthy in the long term for people who are either at a good weight or are underweight—and many cancer patients become underweight.

For these reasons, intermittent fasting is considered a better choice as a form of using diet to reduce cancer risk. In terms of cancer protection, IF:

- stimulates ketosis—which helps prevent obesity, a known cancer risk, and also slows the growth of tumors because cancer cells cannot get energy effectively from ketones.

- limits anabolic (growth) processes—which is important with a disease where cells are growing uncontrolled.

- reduces chronic inflammation—which can cause damage to cells and so increase the risk of cancer.

- increases autophagy—which stimulates damaged cell destruction.

- decreases insulin and increases insulin sensitivity more quickly than CR—which matters because increased levels of insulin are associated with cancer risk.

Research with rats has shown that tumor formation can be blocked with alternate-day fasting. And a test tube study of cancer cells showed that IF made chemotherapy more effective and that it was as effective as chemotherapy in delaying the growth of tumors (Link, 2018a).

Specifically for women, one research study showed that chemotherapy combined with fasting slowed the progression of breast cancer, melanoma, and other skin cancer (Griffith, 2017).

Breast cancer is a type of cancer that is particularly associated with obesity, the body's fat composition, nutrition, and exercise; and intermittent fasting has been shown to be very effective in reducing this cancer risk. We also know that estrogen is a major factor in terms of breast cancer. Insulin interacts a lot with estrogen, and too much body fat increases insulin production. Early research results indicate that intermittent fasting can be effective because it reduces fat and insulin levels (Piersol, 2020).

Reduced Side Effects of Chemotherapy and Radiation

Chemotherapy is a cancer treatment that uses toxic chemicals to kill fast-growing cancer cells. Chemotherapy drugs do not target healthy cells, which grow less slowly, but damage to healthy cells can be a side effect.

One of the reasons healthy cells can be damaged is that some chemotherapy drugs increase levels of blood glucose, which is an easy source of energy for cancer cells. And so, researchers experimented with using intermittent fasting to keep blood glucose down.

Working with mice, they tested a protocol of two to three days of intermittent fasting prior to chemotherapy. The results were positive. Mice who fasted had less damage to healthy cells (Newcomb, 2017).

Insulin and IF

Whenever you eat, your body produces the hormone insulin. Insulin helps glucose enter your cells. If there is more glucose in your blood than your body can use, insulin prompts your body to store it as fat.

When you eat too much, your cells will begin to resist insulin's message to store fat (a condition called insulin resistance). This triggers your body to make more insulin. It is a vicious cycle that can make you sick.

Diabetes is our name for insulin disorders—either too much or too little.

In Chapter 4 I talked about Dr. Jason Fung, a pioneer in the therapeutic use of intermittent fasting to treat diabetes. He has found that intermittent fasting is effective because it decreases blood insulin levels and increases your body's insulin sensitivity, helping to relieve symptoms. It can even put diabetes into remission to the extent that patients no longer need medication.

Research into various modes of intermittent fasting is also promising because all forms of IF studied had the effect of reducing insulin resistance, whether daily eating windows or a schedule of 24-hour fasts (Trumpfeller, 2020a).

But please be aware if you do have pre-diabetes or diabetes, it is very important that you consult a doctor before adopting intermittent fasting, or any other kind of diet.

The benefits of fasting are far-reaching. The more we study it, the more benefits we continue to find.

Chapter 9:

Cellular and Physical Growth

On fasting days, picture your ideal body and remember that your body is dipping into its fat reserve for energy and repairing damaged cells. Let that knowledge encourage and support you. Feel your food addiction weakening its hold on you. –
David Ortner

There are so many ideas that David Ortner touches on in the quote that starts this chapter! He emphasizes what we have been discussing—things like ketosis, weight loss, and hunger. But he does this in the context of the ideas of cellular repair and food addiction, and these ideas do not have to do with breaking down. They have to do with growth.

After all that has been said about ketosis and autophagy, about putting yourself out of anabolism (growth) into a catabolic (break down) phase, you must be wondering… then why did you start the chapter on how IF works talking about body systems, homeostasis, and balance?

You are right. Growth is important too. One of the great strengths of intermittent fasting is that it respects balance between these two processes.

Growth is what I want to focus on in this chapter. So, let's consider cellular and physical growth, and how intermittent fasting benefits these processes.

What Does Food Addiction Have to Do With It?

In Chapter 11, I am going to talk about diet and how to build a healthy, balanced diet that supports a fasting lifestyle. Food addiction is the reverse of that.

David Ortner, who is quoted at the start of the chapter, is the author of nearly a dozen books. He has written several books on 5:2 intermittent fasting. However, he has also written many books on Paleo, Keto, juice cleansing, and the sugar detox diet.

It is true that the 5:2 style of intermittent fasting Ortner promotes tells you that you can eat whatever you want on non-fasting days. But clearly, Ortner is not an advocate of unhealthy eating.

This is where the idea of food addiction comes in.

The International Review of Neurobiology defines food addiction (FA) as "hedonic eating behavior involving the consumption of highly palatable foods (i.e., foods high in salt, fat, and sugar) in quantities beyond homeostatic energy requirements" (Food Addiction - an Overview, n.d.).

There's that idea of homeostasis. If you have a food addiction, you get pleasure from overindulging in food that, in large quantities, is bad for you. This problem is compounded by the fact that most of the addictive foods we are surrounded with today are either snacks that encourage us to eat between meals, or prepackaged food that has been engineered to make us want more: chips, cookies and cake, pizza, burgers, French fries… The list goes on!

There is discussion in the medical community about whether food is truly addictive, in the same way as, say, opioids. But there is agreement about the fact that much manufactured and processed food contains extra amounts of things that trigger the pleasure center of your brain, making you want more.

The result is overeating—not only eating big meals, but also taking in food throughout your waking hours. This leads to a host of health problems, and possibly obesity. If you only stop eating for the eight or so hours while you are asleep, you are in a state of too much growth. Your body is out of balance.

Intermittent fasting is a way to break this cycle.

Healthy Growth

I have focused on ketosis and autophagy as processes that stimulate your body to break down stored fat for food and break down and clean up damaged, diseased, or abnormal cells. The other side of this coin is the role these processes play in triggering healthy growth.

So far, I have been talking about ketosis and autophagy as either/or processes, turning catabolism on or off. Clearly, the body is more complex than that.

Increases in Stem Cells

I talked earlier about the cycle of a cell's life and death. When a cell dies, it is regenerated—replaced with a healthy new cell.

As reported in a study from the Massachusetts Institute of Technology (MIT), cells in the body gradually lose the ability to regenerate. The MIT researchers specifically studied intestinal cells in mice. What they found is that a 24-hour fast, which stimulates ketogenesis, also triggers increased regeneration of stem cells. And the same effect was seen in both young and old mice. (Trafton, 2018).

Stem cells are the basic cells from which all specialized cells are created. The MIT researchers found that when fasting flips the metabolic switch to tell cells to start getting energy from stored fat, stem cell regeneration is also stimulated. In fact, the stem cells' ability to regenerate was doubled.

The study focused specifically on intestinal stem cells, which is interesting because these cells—which regenerate every five days—are an important part of the digestive process. Slower regeneration impairs your ability to digest food and eliminate waste products.

The MIT study followed up earlier research from Valter Longo's lab at USC. Longo and his team demonstrated that prolonged fasting had a twofold effect (Wu, 2014):

- It protected against immune system damage from chemotherapy.

- It stimulated the immune system to regenerate, growing more new white blood cells.

This effect was found in mice who went without food for two to four days a week over a period lasting for six months, and validated in a human clinical trial.

Perhaps this effect of long-term fasting is the basis of that proverb about fasting until you are well.

Mitochondria Repair

Aging is a process of the body slowing down. Digestion slows down. Our ability to use energy slows down. Cellular regeneration slows down. Mitochondrial repair, like an improved immune system, is another way that fasting helps alleviate this process.

Mitochondria are a part of the cell. Their job is to use nutrients to produce energy.

You may have heard of mitochondria in the context of DNA. People get all of their mitochondrial DNA from their mother, which is why it can be used to trace genetic history.

As we age, our mitochondria become less efficient in creating the energy your cells need to function.

Different cells have different numbers of mitochondria. For instance, muscle cells have a lot because they use a lot of energy. However, all human cells except red blood cells contain at least some mitochondria. One of their roles is to break down nutrients and turn them into energy.

Intermittent fasting is now known to support mitochondrial functioning.

Let me digress for a moment to introduce something called adenosine triphosphate, or ATP. ATP is composed of adenosine and three phosphate groups. It allows energy to be transferred into a cell. It does this by releasing one of its three phosphate groups.

When this happens, ATP becomes ADP (adenosine diphosphate). ADP cannot transfer energy to the cell. However, the mitochondria in the cell are able to recharge the ADP, turning it back into ATP, ready for use again.

Evidence from a Harvard study showed that intermittent fasting stimulated the repair of mitochondrial networks, which get fragmented and less effective as we age (Hodapp, n.d.).

Fasting has also been shown to increase mitochondrial biogenesis, or the process of increasing the number of mitochondria in a cell (Fasting and Mitochondrial Health, n.d.).

Improved Gut Health

Research shows that what you eat dramatically affects the composition of your gut microbiome (Stuck, n.d.). Now we are learning that fasting and when you eat affects this microbiome as well.

Gut health—the health of your digestive system—depends on the diversity of the trillions of microorganisms that live in your gut and help it to function. For example, one of the things that it does is form a barrier that keeps toxins and diseases from entering your body.

There is emerging research to show that intermittent fasting can support the health of your gut microbiome (Vetter, 2022):

- In one study, healthy men who fasted during Ramadan were tested at the beginning of the month, at the end of the month, and then once more. At the end of the month, the men had increased levels of a bacteria which has been associated with improved heart health, better mental health, and a lower risk of inflammatory bowel disease and cancer. Significantly, the levels of this bacteria decreased when the men stopped fasting.

- Another study of men who followed the 16:8 plan found that overall microbiome diversity increased, as well as a specific increase in levels of two bacteria linked to improved metabolism and less obesity.

Your body naturally repairs your gut barrier when you sleep at night; however, one hypothesis based on this research is that fasting for longer periods of time increases this benefit.

If your gut barrier is weakened, contents of the digestive system can enter your body before they are finished being processed for use. Some of the health problems associated with a weakened gut barrier are Crohn's Disease, Irritable Bowel Syndrome (IBS), and leaky gut syndrome (which can cause diarrhea, joint pain, bloating, skin problems, and fatigue).

There is also evidence of the various benefits of different types of intermittent fasting (Stuck, n.d.):

- One mouse study found that alternate day 24-hour fasting improved something called bacterial clearance. It turns out that good bacteria need food less often than bad bacteria, and so the 24-hour fast gave time for the number of good bacteria to increase.

- Another mouse study looked at the 16:8 fasting protocol. It found that even when they were given the same type and amount of food, the mice that were not following the 16:8 protocol gained weight, and that weight gain was associated with a very different microbial balance in stool samples from the two groups of mice.

And one final study I would like to mention was done at Imperial College London. It found a correlation between intermittent fasting and an increased ability for mice to recover from nerve damage (London, 2022). Fasting led to a 50% increase in an antioxidant compound which is needed for nerve regeneration, and which is present in humans as well as in mice.

Many of the studies mentioned here did involve mice rather than human subjects. But their results strongly suggest a similar potential for humans to benefit from intermittent fasting's strengthening of the gut microbiome.

Increased Human Growth Hormone (HGH)

Human growth hormone (HGH) has many purposes. It stimulates children to grow. In adults, it is a foundation of good health because it stimulates the body to maintain organs and tissues in good repair and helps you to recover from injury and illness. HGH is also one of the things that declines as we age.

Like Muslims who follow Ramadan, many people who follow the Mormon faith incorporate fasting into their lives. As a result, the Intermountain Medical Center in Utah is uniquely able to investigate the health benefits of fasting.

In one study, HGH was shown to increase on average by nearly 2,000% in men and by 1,300% in women during a 24-hour fasting period (Study Finds Routine Periodic Fasting Is Good for Your Health, and Your Heart, 2011).

Other research points to links between intermittent fasting and HGH. Among the findings (Youplushealth, 2020):

- A 3-day fast increased HGH levels more than 300%, and after a week, levels had continued to rise to 1,250%.

- Body fat, and especially belly fat, lowers HGH production.

- Intermittent fasting helps reduce body fat, which helps increase HGH.

- Intermittent fasting reduces insulin in the blood, which helps increase HGH.

Returning to the idea of metabolic balance, by fasting your body stimulates the catabolic processes of ketosis and autophagy, and at the same time stimulates an increase in HGH. HGH is vital to the anabolic process of normal repair and recovery from illness and injury.

Decreased Androgen Markers in Women

Androgens are sex hormones. The one you are probably familiar with is the most common one: testosterone. Both men and women have androgens, but men have more of them.

What do androgens do? They promote healthy bone density, the production of red blood cells, muscle development, sexuality, and puberty. In men they are responsible for face and body hair growth, deepening of the voice, and the development of sperm. In women, they are responsible for the growth of underarm and pubic hair, help regulate menstruation and pregnancy, and protect against osteoporosis.

Your androgen levels naturally decline as you get older. And androgen markers measure the amounts of these hormones in your blood.

One emerging area of research concerns the impact of intermittent fasting on reproductive health. A study published in 2022 had several findings, which differed for men and for women (Cienfuegos et al., 2022):

- Intermittent fasting, especially when eating periods ended by 4:00 p.m., decreased androgen markers in premenopausal women with obesity but increased markers for the protein, SHBG, that transports it.

- Intermittent fasting also reduced testosterone levels in young men who were lean and physically active, but did not affect levels of SHBG.

These are very preliminary, inconclusive results. But they do show that there is a correlation between fasting and androgen.

There is more to learn. For instance, intermittent fasting may have an effect on polycystic ovary syndrome (PCOS), which is a condition that can affect women of any age or ethnicity. PCOS is the result of an overabundance of male hormones and lack of female hormones. It causes ovarian cysts, irregular or missed periods, and excess facial and body hair.

One thing we know is that being overweight is a factor in PCOS, so a lifestyle that supports healthy weight is beneficial. An excess of insulin is another factor that is implicated with PCOS, and a lifestyle that helps regulate insulin levels is beneficial. And in fact, intermittent fasting has been shown to reduce androgens and help relieve PCOS symptoms (Cellante, 2020).

Are you dealing with PCOS? Digestive issues? Chronic pain? If you are, look to intermittent fasting for answers.

100

Part 4:

How to Intermittent Fast

Chapter 10:

Mental/Physical Preparation and Training

During a fast you will find out if it is you that controls your thoughts or if it is your thoughts that control you. –Author unknown

I hope by now you are convinced that intermittent fasting offers a whole range of benefits that you would like to bring into your life.

I have been presenting IF as a simple way to become healthier in many different ways. It is. It will also be easier—and more effective—if you prepare.

Let's talk about that now.

Adjust Your View of Eating

Yes, I am talking about your relationship with food.

Your relationship with food—how you handle decisions about what you eat—has a huge impact on both your overall health and on how challenging or easy it will be for you to adopt an intermittent fasting lifestyle.

To start, let me ask you some questions:

- What is your food routine? Do you think that breakfast is the most important meal of the day, and that everyone needs "three square meals" a day? Are you a grazer, eating two or three meals but also snacking in the morning, afternoon, and evening? How often do you cook and how often eat out?

- Do you think that you eat too much, or too little? Does your weight yoyo up and down? Or are you one of those folks who weighs pretty much the same thing you always have?

- What do you eat? What do you like to eat? Are they the same?

- Do you pick up the same things at the grocery store all the time? Do you follow the latest food or diet fads? If you are going to a party, do you ever find yourself worrying about what you are going to eat?

- Are there some foods you simply crave? Is it the same thing all the time?

- How much do you think about food—specifically about what you are going to eat?

Develop a Good Relationship With Food

People who have a good relationship with food are healthy and able to enjoy eating without letting food (or thoughts of food) dominate their life.

And, as you are keenly aware if you are experiencing or have gone through menopause, this is a relationship that changes over time.

There are many reasons for this. One is metabolism.

Remember being a kid and able to eat pretty much anything you wanted without gaining weight? Remember how once you were an adult you had to learn to moderate how much you ate because you simply were not burning up as much energy as you did before?

According to a study I read in the magazine Science, our metabolism is at its peak when we are about a year old, which is why babies need to eat every hour or so. From then our metabolism goes down by about 3% each year until we are 20. It stays relatively stable for decades, but then starts to go down again by about 1% a year when we are in our 60s (Stenson, 2021). At each stage, you need to adjust your relationship with food.

If you are a woman in your 50s you are probably thinking, "Come on. My metabolism changed when I was pregnant. And now there's menopause. What about that?"

I was surprised that the article said that, in fact, pregnancy and menopause do not cause a change in your metabolism. But that does not mean they do not cause a change in your relationship with food!

Pregnant women get food cravings. That is real. And even if your metabolism is the same, as I mentioned earlier, women going through menopause on average gain five to eight percent of their pre-menopausal body weight in the first two years.

Clearly, there are factors that affect our relationship with food. These are emotional, social, cultural, and physical.

You know you have a bad relationship with food if you are stressed about what you eat. Here are some signs you may recognize:

- you are always on a diet

- you need to count calories in order to maintain your desired weight

- you think eating is a guilty pleasure, or have a list of foods you need to avoid

- sometimes you just binge on food

- you worry about what you are going to eat when you are going to a party or out to dinner

When I learned about this it made me realize that having a bad relationship with food is about far more than being the weight you want. And I wanted to know how to improve my relationship with food.

It can be tough to change your eating habits, and tough to stick with a new plan when you are going through hard times. But there are things that you can do; and success will help you keep with it. Here is what I learned.

Get a Good Night's Sleep

We know that, on average, people who get only four good hours of sleep a night eat 550 extra calories a day. This is because your stomach makes two appetite hormones, one that tells you that you are hungry and the other that says you have had enough. When you are sleep deprived, your hunger hormone rises and your sated hormone falls (Peeke, 2010).

Eating 550 extra calories adds up to 3,850 calories a week. For the average person, this is the equivalent of gaining a pound each week.

Here are things you can do to get a better night's sleep:

- Try to go to bed at the same time every night. Sure, there will be times that this will change, but keeping to a regular schedule is soothing and you will find it easier to fall asleep.

- Unplug. Put down the phone and turn off the video.

- Relax. For example, you might try simply deep breathing or telling your body to relax from your toes to the top of your head.

- Do your best to de-stress. It is hard to fall asleep when your mind is stuck on a hamster wheel of thought. Try meditation, yoga, or journaling.

Learn How to Recognize When You Are Hungry

This is a challenge if, like many people in the Western world, you have rarely—if ever—felt real hunger pangs.

When you are hungry, your stomach growls. You may feel like your energy is down. Your blood sugar will dip, too, which is why people with pre-diabetes or diabetes should talk with their doctor before starting to fast.

All too often, however, your mind tells you that you want something to eat when you are simply bored or anxious or unhappy and want something to make you feel good. Learn to recognize when this is happening so you can redirect. Have a glass of water, or eat a piece of fruit instead of a snack bar.

There are lots of reasons you might eat when you are not hungry. Here are a few:

- You see that the food is there, so you "just have one."

- You are in a social situation where someone is pushing you to eat.

- You are in the habit of eating in a certain environment—this could be when you are watching TV, at a football game, or spend a lot of time in the kitchen preparing family meals.

- You are stressed or feeling emotional.

Be Mindful About What You Are Eating

I am not talking about dieting. I am talking about awareness.

When you are shopping, read food labels so that you know what is actually in the food that you eat. Do as much shopping as you can on the perimeter of the store; that is where the least processed food items are. It can be helpful to have a shopping list.

Choose to eat things that make you feel well—both mentally and physically.

Eat at the table, don't simply stand there in the kitchen. Focus on the moment. Slow down and enjoy each bite. Chew. No, not like Fletcherism; what I mean is to enjoy the flavor and not just gulp it down.

Start with a smaller portion and take smaller bites. Then wait a few minutes before taking more. It takes a little while for your food to get to your stomach and the "I've had enough" hormone to kick in.

Take Small Steps and Be Realistic About What You Can Do

It is like that old adage: "How do you eat a bear? One bite at a time."

Start with what is most manageable for you, whether it is changing your sleep routine, changing portion sizes, or starting to read food labels. The important thing is to start.

Do not give up if you miss a bite. This is not an all-or-nothing process. You can start again.

Don't Forget the Supplements

Depending on your diet, you may take supplements to make sure you are getting enough micronutrients and electrolytes. Vegetarians or vegans, for example, must often consider these.

When you decide to try intermittent fasting it will be important to evaluate any supplements you are taking and choose an IF protocol that accommodates your dietary needs. This is especially important because some supplements are supposed to be taken with food and others are not.

The same is true of some medications, and you should consult your doctor or pharmacists about this before starting to fast. But let me talk about supplements.

Because fasting is about when you eat, not restricting what you eat, it is possible to fast and get good nutrition. This is only true, of course, if you are eating a healthy, well-balanced diet (to be discussed in the next chapter).

If it is possible, I recommend taking your supplements with your meals. In this way it will be easy to avoid inadvertently breaking your fast.

Any supplements that have calories will break a fast. As you know, one of the goals of intermittent fasting is to gain a state of ketosis. Any calories you consume during a fasting period will prevent ketosis.

Supplements that are best absorbed with food:

- amino acid or amino acid combinations, such as BCAAs

- chromium and vanadium

- curcumin or turmeric

- fat-soluble vitamins such as vitamins A, D, and K

- fatty acids, such as omega-3 fatty acids or medium-chain triglycerides (MCTs)

- iodine

- krill oil or mega krill complex

- kelp powder or potassium iodide

- magnesium

- protein powders, which typically contain >100 calories per scoop

- sweetened electrolyte drink powders or effervescent tablets

- sweetened gummy or chewable supplements

- supplements which contain sweeteners or additional ingredients, such as fruit juice, cane sugar, or starches

- zinc and copper

There are some supplements that you can take without food and that will probably not put you into ketosis.

Supplements to take without food:

- iron

- tyrosine

- folic acid

- probiotics

- water-soluble vitamins, such as vitamins B and C

There are also a few supplements you might eat before a fast in order to help suppress your appetite and also promote your transition into ketosis. These are:

- soluble fiber, which will help you feel more full and less hungry

- omega-3 fatty acids, which help reduced your appetite and feelings of hunger

- medium-chain triglycerides (MCTs), which increase metabolism and promote ketosis

- curcumin, which decreases insulin resistance

Physical Training to Enhance Your Results

We discussed the likely role of fasting in the evolution of humankind and how, when they were hungry and forced to fast until their next meal, our prehistoric ancestors were at a peak of physical readiness and mental clarity.

It is safe to exercise when you are fasting, and in fact exercise can boost its benefits. For instance, we talked about how exercise can increase the amount of fat you will burn.

But, especially if you are following a protocol with an extended fast, there are some important concerns that you should consider:

- Long-term fasting can cause your metabolism to slow down.

- You may become fatigued, which will affect your performance.

- Extended fasting may result in a loss of muscle mass because your body will start to use protein for energy when you have depleted stored fat.

Guidelines for how to exercise will depend on the IF protocol you choose to follow and how much exercise you are used to doing. What you want to do is plan to exercise when your body has enough energy (whether from a recent meal or while you are burning fat).

The period when you are first fasting is not the best time to ramp up your exercise schedule. When you start a fasting regimen, stick with your normal type of exercise. Consider ramping up once your body is adjusted to fasting.

If you are following a protocol like 16:8 or 12:12, choose a fasting window and exercise time that is best for your schedule and exercise goals. If you fast for a full 24 hours or more, however, it is a good idea to limit exercise to things that are low-intensity. Walking, gentle Pilates, or a less vigorous form of yoga are good choices.

The type of exercise you do will be a major factor in deciding the timing of exercise and meals.

- A low-intensity workout, Pilates, yoga, or barre: You should be able to do this type of workout during most types of IF, especially if you want to exercise while you are in the fasted state.

- High intensity interval training (HIIT): People often choose this type of intense workout with the goal of losing weight and burning fat. If HIIT is already part of your exercise schedule, you may be able to continue while you are fasting—especially if your workout is 30 minutes or less. However, depending on where you are in the IF cycle, you may lack the energy you need to perform to your expected level, or you may find that you are losing muscle mass or driving down your blood sugar level.

- Strength-training/weight lifting: It is best to do this type of exercise during your eating window because your goal is to build up muscle. If you exercise like this in a fasted state, your body may start to use protein instead of stored fat for fuel. If you do work out during your fasting window, follow your workout with a meal that has plenty of protein and complex carbohydrates.

- Moderate morning run: It is okay to run in a fasted state, and you can wait a few hours before eating unless you feel dizzy and weak.

In general, it is a good idea to exercise earlier in the day because that fits well with the body's natural circadian rhythm. However, it may be better for you to exercise in the middle of the day or right after work. That is okay. What you want to do is avoid working out late in the day because this will make it harder for you to get a good night's sleep.

Always pay attention to your body. Drink water to stay hydrated and replenish electrolytes lost. Coconut water may be a better choice for this than a sports drink or Gatorade that have a lot of sugar.

If you are dehydrated or have low blood sugar, you may feel weak and dizzy. If you choose an especially rigorous form of fasting, you may not feel able to exercise as vigorously as you do when you are eating. The important thing is to respect what your body is telling you and do what feels good.

Chapter 11:

Building a Balanced Diet Plan

One of the reasons intermittent fasting can work is that it reconnects you with what hunger feels like. –Chris Mohr

Chris Mohr is a football player. He was starting punter for his 4 years with the Crimson Tide at the University of Alabama and played 15 years for the Tampa Bay Buccaneers. Chris Mohr knows something about fitness. And he advocates fasting as part of a balanced diet plan.

Let's talk about what it means to eat a healthy, balanced diet when you are intermittent fasting.

How and What to Eat

I have emphasized that intermittent fasting is concerned with when you eat. The purpose is to create a continuous period of time—at least eight hours—during which you do not eat at all. That is the source of fasting's benefits.

The ultimate goal is to make fasting a routine part of your life.

Choosing the Right IF Protocol

One of the best things to me about intermittent fasting is its flexibility. There is no one best way to do it. And you can make changes to your protocol as your life changes.

115

There are basically four types of protocol that you might follow. As discussed in Chapter 3, there are some programs, such as the Juice Fast, that allow you to ingest minimal calories on so-called fasting days. But these are CR diets, not true fasts. I mention them because they can be a way for you to ease into true fasting.

Throughout this book I have also discussed longer periods of fasting, such as protocols used by Dr. Fung to treat patients with diabetes. But this type of extended fasting is not generally considered intermittent fasting. It cannot be sustained and it requires medical supervision.

As a rule of thumb, fasting for more than 36 hours is not considered intermittent fasting.

In this section of the book, I'll discuss the pros and cons of the five major IF protocols to help you choose the one for you. Three of these involve daily fasting and two involve a weekly fasting schedule.

12:12

The 12:12 IF protocol is to eat in a 12-hour window and fast for 12 hours.

This may be the easiest introduction to intermittent fasting and the easiest protocol to stick with. If you routinely finish dinner before 8:00 p.m. and simply stop eating after dinner, you can fast overnight, and eat breakfast at or after 8:00 a.m.

If snacking is a problem for you, this is a good way to start because you can practice with a relatively small awake fasting window.

However, you may not get the maximum benefit from IF with 12:12 because, if you are overweight and prone to overeating, ketosis may not kick in.

16:8

The 16:8 IF protocol has a 16-hour fasting window.

On average, people start to experience ketosis after about 12 hours. That makes 16:8 a very popular form of IF that, like 12:12, is relatively easy to fit into a busy lifestyle.

One simple way to get started with 16:8 is meal skipping. If you finish dinner by 8:00 p.m. and do not break your fast until the next day at lunch, sometime after 12 p.m., you will have fasted for 16 hours.

This protocol is especially easy for people who do not like to eat breakfast. In fact, some people who do not eat breakfast and also do not snack between meals are actually following a 16:8 IF protocol without realizing it.

But if you are someone who wakes up hungry and needs the energy you get from breakfast, 16:8 can be tough. If this is you and you want to try 16:8, you may find that the chapter on diet has ideas that can help make 16:8 work for you.

23/1 (OMAD)

One meal a day is the third of the daily IF protocols. You can eat whatever you want in the one-hour window when you eat your one meal each day.

The Warrior Diet is similar, but has a longer four-hour eating window.

OMAD is a very simple protocol, but it can be hard to follow. It is also very important to combine this type of IF with a healthy, well-balanced diet. Otherwise, you will get sick.

People who suffer from health issues such as diabetes should consult their doctor before starting OMAD.

5:2

When you follow the 5:2 IF protocol you eat normally five days a week. On two days, you eat only 500 or 600 calories. In order to get the benefit of ketosis and autophagy, you will need to consume your calories in a restricted window of time rather than grazing throughout the day.

You should have at least one eating day between your two fasting days.

Eat Stop Eat is similar to 5:2 except that you do not eat anything for your two 24-hour fasting periods.

If you want to adopt 5:2 IF, you may want to start with a weekly 24-hour fast.

Alternate Day

The Alternate Day IF protocol is straightforward. You fast for 24 hours every other day. As with 5:2, there is a version of Alternate Day fasting where you eat a limited number of calories on fasting days and a version where you do not eat at all.

This is the most rigorous IF protocol and probably will not fit into everyone's lifestyle.

All this being said, how do you choose? Here are some considerations:

- If you are new to fasting it is a good idea to start with a relatively easy program and work your way up to something more rigorous if you want.

- If you have a bad relationship with food and know that hunger is going to be a challenge for you, read the section on diet carefully and consider changing your diet before you start fasting.

- Be sure to choose an IF protocol that will work with your busy life.

- What are your health goals? For instance:

    o Do you want to lose weight? If so, a longer fast can be a good choice because you will simply have less time to consume calories. But be sure to eat a healthy diet the rest of the time.

    o How important is it for you to increase or maintain lean muscle mass? The shorter daily protocols are a good choice for this.

A word of caution. IF is not healthy for growing children, or for women who are pregnant or breastfeeding. It can be dangerous for someone who has had an eating disorder or is underweight. And it should only be followed with medical supervision if you suffer from a blood sugar problem such as diabetes.

That being said, one big challenge when you practice IF is to avoid overeating and binge eating. If you have a bad relationship with food, it can be easy to let your eating get out of control in your eating window.

Choosing the Right Foods to Eat

Let me repeat as I have throughout this book, intermittent fasting does not prescribe the food you eat. For many, the fact that you can eat whatever you want is a real selling point.

However, if you want to make the most of IF, you need to eat a healthy, well-balanced diet that supplies all the nutrients your body needs.

Why? Because fasting and diet work together:

- What you eat affects how much fat your body stores.

- Your diet determines how much energy you have throughout the day.

- A good diet helps your digestive system work well, and as you know the effects of fasting flow from there.

- A healthy diet also promotes many of the same health benefits you can gain through IF, and combining IF with a good diet plan will get you more bang for your bucks.

There are a number of published plans that describe a healthy diet. I am sure you are familiar with the basic rules:

- Try to eat whole grains instead of refined grains.

- When choosing protein, limit red and processed meat in favor of fish, poultry, beans, or nuts.

- Eat a colorful variety of fruits and vegetables, but avoid too many potatoes since potatoes have a lot of starch that increases blood sugar.

- Limit your use of butter and trans fat, and use more plant oils.

- Drink water. Limit fruit juice and other drinks that are high in sugar.

- Limit milk and dairy to two servings a day.

Foods that are nutrient-dense are particularly good choices when you are intermittent fasting. These include fruits and vegetables, whole grains, beans, nuts and seeds, lean proteins, and dairy.

Foods that are high in fiber have more bulk, which will help you feel fuller during a fast. Foods that are high in fiber are also good for digestion, helping to keep you regular. High fiber foods include whole foods and grains, and cruciferous vegetables like cauliflower, broccoli, and brussels sprouts.

It is important to stay hydrated. Drinking water is also a good way to alleviate hunger pangs.

Avocado is a healthy choice. Avocados are high in calories, but they also have a lot of unsaturated fat. This is helpful because unsaturated fats postpone the release of the hunger hormone.

The general food guidelines recommend not eating too many potatoes, but what I will call unprocessed potatoes can be a good choice leading into a fast because they are very filling. By unprocessed I mean potatoes that are boiled or baked, not chips or fries.

When you are choosing protein, fish and seafood can be a good choice. They are relatively low in calories and provide lots of protein, healthy fats, and vitamin D. Beans and legumes are another good source of protein, and are also a good source of carbohydrates for energy to support your fast. Eggs, too, are a great source of protein and are a much lower-calorie and more filling breakfast than cereal or a bagel.

Nuts and seeds are foods to consider. They are high in calories so you do not want to eat too many. But they also have high levels of healthy fat.

Berries are a great source of important nutrients, and there is evidence that people who eat blueberries and strawberries that contain a lot of flavonoids gain less body mass over time (Rizzo, 2022).

And finally, probiotics. These are foods that support a healthy gut microbiome. Foods that are rich in probiotics include yogurt and kefir, sauerkraut and pickles, tempeh (fermented soybean), kimchi, and miso.

When you are experimenting with changing your diet, give new foods a try. You may find that you like them.

Macros... Micros... Huh?

We're talking about nutrients here. Macronutrients are what your body needs in relatively large amounts. Micronutrients are essential but needed in much smaller amounts. Macronutrients are carbohydrates, proteins, and fats. Vitamins and minerals are micronutrients.

I saw something interesting on a website written by doctor of functional and integrative medicine Will Cole: "Your body is not a calorie counter. It is a chemistry lab, and intermittent fasting resets the beautiful biochemistry lab otherwise known as your metabolism" (The Chalkboard Editorial Team, 2021).

Macronutrients and micronutrients are the materials of this lab.

Dr. Cole is emphasizing one of the themes of intermittent fasting. IF is not about calorie restriction; it is about restricting the frequency with which you eat.

Combined with a healthy diet, IF can lead to healthy weight loss. And it will help you sustain a healthy weight.

With that in mind, let me share a few general guidelines to consider when you are deciding what and how to eat while you are intermittent fasting.

Getting the Right Kinds of Fat

Despite dieting advice that tells you to eliminate or restrict fat in your diet, your body needs fat.

Fat is important for your brain.

It also speeds up your metabolism, helps regulate blood sugar, helps you absorb vitamins, and makes you feel full. In these ways fat helps protect you from diabetes, obesity, and cardiovascular diseases.

However, there are three different kinds of fat, and you need to eat the good ones. The three kinds of fat are: unsaturated, saturated, and trans fats.

Unsaturated fats are fats that come from plants and are liquid at room temperature. Without going into too much chemical detail, these good fats improve your level of blood cholesterol, help your heart beat steadily, and ease inflammation.

You will find unsaturated fats in vegetable oils, avocados, cheese, seeds and nuts, whole eggs, fish, full fat yogurt, and dark chocolate.

Saturated fats are fats that come from red meat, dairy products, and tropical oils such as coconut and palm oil. Saturated fats may increase your risk of stroke or heart disease. However. we do need some saturated fat in our diet. These fats contribute to the health of your liver, skin, brain, and immune system.

What your body does not need, and what you should actively avoid, are trans fats. Even in small quantities trans fats raise the level of LDL cholesterol in your blood, significantly increasing your risk of cardiovascular disease.

Trans fats are found mostly in fried and processed foods, a product of hydrogenated oil. The U.S. Food and Drug Administration (FDA) has required manufacturers to eliminate trans fats from food products. But you may still see hydrogenated oil listed on food labels. If you do, do not eat that food.

Getting Enough Protein

As with every nutrient, you need to eat protein, but not too much.

Proteins do many things for our bodies:

- They are called building blocks, the nutrient your body uses for growth, maintenance, and repair.

- They are a source of energy.

- They are involved in the production of some hormones.

- In the form of enzymes, they fuel chemical reactions in the body.

- Proteins such as hemoglobin transport and store nutrients throughout the body.

- Other proteins function in the immune system to create antibodies.

On average, a healthy diet should include between 10%–35% of daily calories in protein. This wide range reflects the fact that the amount of protein you need depends on how active you are. There are a number of online nutrition calculators you can use to figure out your individual protein needs.

Most people do not need to worry about eating too much protein (unless they suffer from kidney disease). On the other hand, if you do not eat enough protein your body will start to break down muscle tissue to derive the proteins that it needs. This is usually not a problem for people living in developed countries.

However, our bodies cannot store protein. Proteins do break down in the body, and some part of this is excreted. But part of it will be converted to glucose and stored in the body as fat.

Getting the Right Amount of Carbs

Carbohydrates, especially complex carbohydrates, are another important component of nutrition. As is the case with fat, there are diets based on cutting carbs from your diet. And as with fat, it is important to take this all with a grain of salt.

Complex carbohydrates are found in unprocessed food from plants, things like: whole grains, beans, white and sweet potatoes, carrots, asparagus, apples, oranges, and berries. Simple carbs are found in fruits, milk and milk products, and processed and refined sugar.

It is healthy to limit the simple carbohydrates you eat, but your body uses both kinds.

Carbohydrates are chains of sugar molecules. Complex carbs are longer chains that take longer to digest. They are converted into glucose that the body uses for energy. The shorter chains of simple carbohydrates break down more quickly, and so they deliver glucose more quickly. However, many simple carbs derived from processed foods are low in nutrients and should be avoided.

If you have diabetes or prediabetes, it is especially important for you to control your carbohydrate consumption. There are lots of effective ways to do this. Here are a few:

- Do not drink too many sugary drinks.

- Avoid ultra-processed food, things like instant soup or chicken nuggets. The challenge, of course, is that these food products are cheap and easy.

- Eat more whole than refined grain food (bread, rice, etc.). You might consider substituting spaghetti squash or zucchini noodles for pasta. Or use cauliflower rice.

- There are some simple ways to limit bread in your diet. You can make lettuce wraps instead of burritos or burgers. Or make an open-faced sandwich.

- Try to eat fruit instead of drinking fruit juice since fruit juice has little fiber and is high in simple sugar.

- Avoid chips and other salty, savory snacks and try instead to snack on things like nuts, cheese, or eggs.

- Look for lower-carb food at breakfast, perhaps choosing eggs or a low-carb cereal instead of sugary cereal or a bagel.

When you transition to a healthier diet, as with any new thing, there may be some trial and error. Start slow and be patient with yourself.

Chapter 12:

Popular Diet Programs

Intermittent fasting is a lifestyle. It isn't something that you start today and then end when you get to some arbitrary "goal weight." Something you start and then stop is a DIET. Intermittent fasting isn't a diet — as I said, it's a lifestyle. –Gin Stephens

Gin Stephens is the author of *Delay, Don't Deny: Living an Intermittent Fasting Lifestyle.* She has herself followed this lifestyle since 2014, and at the same time lost more than 80 lbs.

In the previous chapter I talked about the importance of a balanced diet and how eating a balanced diet contributes to the effectiveness of intermittent fasting. However, I know that many people who are successfully following certain diet plans, especially if they are trying to reach a particular weight loss goal, will want to continue with their diet too.

You can certainly combine intermittent fasting with a diet that is working for you.

It is important to understand that both dieting and fasting can have a big impact on your body's metabolism. It will be an adjustment. But one that is well worth it.

Let me also mention that, whatever diet you follow, it is important to make sure that you are still getting the minimum daily amount of all the nutrients you need.

If this is you, you may want to start intermittent fasting too. So let me briefly discuss some popular diets and IF.

High-Protein Diet

In Chapter 11 I said that, depending on your level of activity, you need to eat 10%–35% of your daily calories in the form of protein. A high-protein diet starts within this range, with 20% of your daily calories coming from protein. These diets also restrict carbs, and sometimes vegetables.

Some popular high protein diets are Atkins and the Zone.

High-protein diets work for weight loss because when you eat fewer carbohydrates your body will run out of blood sugar more quickly when you are fasting.

I discussed some of the risks of eating too much protein in the earlier chapter. In addition, you may actually gain weight since many sources of protein are high calorie. Other people find that a high-protein diet causes GI problems (either constipation or diarrhea).

Low-Carb Diet

As the name indicates, a low-carb diet restricts the amount of carbs you eat, emphasizing foods that are high in protein and fat. There are many different low-carb diet plans.

Many people choose a low-carb diet because it lets them eat more of the foods they particularly enjoy. The diet can help you lose weight; however, some people may experience muscle cramps, constipation, or headaches.

If you are following a low-carb diet, pay attention to the types of carbs you consume: You want to emphasize foods that contain the healthier complex carbs.

There is no evidence that a low-carb diet is more effective for weight loss than a well-balanced CR diet. But there is evidence that people who follow a low-carb diet for months or years can develop heart problems, osteoporosis, kidney damage, lipid abnormalities, impaired physical activity; and experience an increased risk of cancer, or even sudden death (Bilsborough & Crowe, 2003).

Low-Fat Diet

People who have gallbladder or pancreas disease should follow a low-fat diet. But it is generally understood that a low-fat diet alone is not enough if your goal is to lose significant weight. Low-fat weight loss diets restrict calories as well as high-fat foods.

As we discussed, fats are an important component of a balanced diet. In fact, dietary guidelines call for you to get as much as 20%–35% of your calories each day from fats. However, you also want to be sure to eat more unsaturated fats, some saturated fats, and no trans fats at all.

Some healthy ways to reduce fat in your diet include:

- Trim fat from meat and remove skin from poultry.

- Eat lots of leafy greens and fruits.

- Give sweet potatoes a try; they are high in nutrition and low in fat.

- Remove fat from soup, gravy, or stew by refrigerating it and removing the hardened fat.

- Avoid frying. Try baking, broiling, and grilling instead.

- Try using yogurt instead of sour cream.

- When you are eating out, avoid fried foods and heavy sauces, and ask for salad dressing on the side.

Mediterranean Diet

The Mediterranean Diet and intermittent fasting work very well together.

The Mediterranean Diet is one of the most well-known and well-regarded diet, ranked as the #1 best diet by U.S. News & World Report in 2022. It is touted for its benefits in terms of weight loss, cancer and diabetes prevention, and heart and brain health.

Rather than focus on calorie intake, the Mediterranean Diet focuses on the foods that you eat—basically the same foods that are typically consumed in countries bordering the Mediterranean Sea. The diet varies, as does the diet in different Mediterranean countries.

The central idea is to enjoy good food in moderation, and to do so in the company of loved ones. Being physically active is also important.

In addition to weight loss, among the benefits of this diet are:

- reduced risk of heart disease (the #1 disease affecting Americans)

- reduced risk of stroke for women

- prevention or amelioration in loss of cognition

- prevention or amelioration of Type 2 diabetes

- amelioration of rheumatoid arthritis

- protection against cancer

- and the diet is even said to help lessen depression

Of course, portion control is up to you. And here are some recommendations for you to follow if you are fasting and following the Mediterranean Diet:

- Eat primarily plant-based or seafood proteins.

- Use extra virgin olive oil as your primary source of fat.

- Use whole grains, fruits, and vegetables.

- Use salt-free seasoning.

- Include some calcium-rich food in your diet every day.

Paleo Diet

Both intermittent fasting and the Paleo Diet arise from our understanding of prehistoric humans. Specifically, the idea of the Paleo Diet is to eat the same foods as did prehistoric man, at the time when food was not routinely available. It is a real-food diet that recommends eating primarily meats, including organ meats, seafood and shellfish, eggs, vegetables, fruits, nuts, and seeds. It may also include some dairy, legumes, and grains.

One advantage of the Paleo Diet is that following it makes it simple to avoid the manufactured food products that are a source of unhealthy eating today.

Among the benefits of this diet are said to be:

- weight loss

- improved mental health and cognition

- better metabolism

- less risk of developing such chronic diseases as cardiovascular disease, diabetes, or obesity

When you are following a Paleo Diet while intermittent fasting, you want to be sure to eat enough during your eating window to support your body well in the fasting period.

Keto Diet

The Keto Diet emphasizes proteins and fats with only a few carbs. The goal is to deplete carbohydrate reserves in order to encourage the body toward ketosis. The big difference between a Keto and low-carb diet is how strict it is; you are supposed to eat 70% of your calories from fat, 20% from protein, and only 10% from carbs. The goal is to put yourself into ketosis.

The Keto Diet can be an effective weight-loss regime, and there are potential benefits that include less acne, reduced risk of cancer and heart disease, improved brain function, fewer seizures, and relief of PCOS symptoms.

However, there are some potential problems. You will eat very few vegetables on this diet, and it can be hard to get all of the nutrients you need. The diet can have side effects which include GI trouble, low energy, vomiting, low iron, kidney stones, and high cholesterol.

There is currently no evidence that Keto and IF are an effective combination. In fact, because both Keto and IF seek to put the body into ketosis, the two together may be too much.

There is a lot to consider if you want to combine intermittent fasting with a specific diet you also follow.

If you feel like you are stuck, you can always mix up your diet plan. And if you are looking to lose the most weight possible, combining keto and IF has been shown to be the most beneficial.

134

Part 5:

Lifestyle Transformation

Chapter 13:

Transforming You in 5 Steps: Your Path and Your Pace 5-Step Program to Finding Success With IF

Everyone has a doctor in him or her; we just have to help it in its work. The natural healing force within each one of us is the greatest force in getting well. Our food should be our medicine. Our medicine should be our food. But to eat when you are sick, is to feed your sickness. —Hippocrates

I introduce the final chapter with this quote from Hippocrates, emphasizing the profound health benefits of the IF lifestyle.

I first heard of intermittent fasting as a weight-loss program. It was the extra weight I had gained during menopause that pushed me to try intermittent fasting. I had tried so many diets in the past that simply did not work. And weight-loss dieting was somewhat of a downer, too.

But intermittent fasting worked.

Then I saw a poster with a quote from an author unknown that sort of sums it up for me: "What if I told you that intermittent fasting was really intermittent eating?"

Yes!

It was only after I had achieved my weight loss goal that I realized, intermittent fasting makes me really feel good, too.

So now, after going over what intermittent fasting is and what it can do for you, I want to share a five-step program you can use to make IF a part of your life.

Step 1: Decide on Your Diet Plan

Intermittent fasting works best when combined with a balanced diet.

If you are like me, you will be starting IF in combination with a weight-loss diet, perhaps High Protein, Low Carb, Low Fat, Mediterranean, Paleo, or Keto. If you do this, evaluate what you are eating to be sure that you get enough macro and micro nutrients every day.

Fasting puts stress on your body. That is the point. So, you want your body to be well-prepared to handle it.

If you are not on a weight-loss diet, you should still evaluate what you are eating. Specifically, plan what to eat before and after each fasting period.

Step 2: Choose the Fasting Method to Start

Which of the many IF protocols makes the most sense for you to use?

Decide if you are going to start with 12:12, 16:8, OMAD, 5:2, Alternate Day, or perhaps even a weekly 24-hour fast.

OMAD may be the easiest way in for you. Perhaps it's 12:12. Or you may be the kind of person who likes to jump-start things and choose to fast the entire day after Thanksgiving dinner.

Do not worry if the protocol you choose ends up not being the right one. Simply choose another.

Step 3: Select Your Starting Point

If you are new to fasting, ease into it. You may not be ready to start fasting right away and, if that is the case, your starting point might be eliminating snacks from what you eat each day.

Or, if you are ready to start with one of the daily plans like 16:8, make a daily plan to gradually decrease your eating window and increase the fasting period.

If you are already on the IF road, perhaps you would like to adopt a more rigorous fasting method, for instance, moving from 16:8 to the Alternate Day. Again, it is okay to take it slowly.

Step 4: Customize a 6-Week Program

Rather than saying, "I am an intermittent faster now and this is what I am going to do for the rest of my life," tell yourself, "I am going to give intermittent fasting a try."

Six weeks is a good amount of time, because if you stick with it for six weeks you will have a chance to really experience the benefits of IF.

Keep a journal that lists each of your goals and metrics that will let you track your progress; for example: weight loss, exercise, or relaxation activity.

When I started IF I was not sure about how to do it, so I looked online and found a lot of ideas. There was one website with hundreds of free templates for different kinds of logs, and another one called FitCoach that had an online quiz that generated a personalized plan for me.

My first log was a series of six charts with seven columns (one for each day) and five rows for breakfast, lunch, dinner, exercise, and relaxation/stress busting. I put a check mark for each meal that I ate, wrote down how I exercised, and what I did to relax.

It felt good to look at my charts and see real progress!

Step 5: Maintain a 40-Day IF Schedule and Chart Your Success

Celebrate your successes after six weeks and evaluate how you did.

How much progress did you make? Did you achieve your goal or goals? Do you have a new goal?

Follow up your success with a 40-day plan. You can use the same chart you started with or create a new one if your IF plan or goals have changed.

And that's it. Let me wish you a bon voyage!

Conclusion

I hope you have enjoyed this exploration of a lifestyle that is such a rewarding influence in the lives of so many.

If you have, please leave a review to share your thoughts with me.

Glossary

16:8: A popular form of intermittent fasting in which you fast for 16 hours each day, and eat in an 8-hour window.

5:2: A form of intermittent fasting developed by Dr. Michael Mosley, also known as the "Fast Diet." It mandates five days of normal calorie intake, with two "fasting" days of 500 calories.

Alternate day fasting (ADF): Eating no calories at all on fasting days, alternating with feast days where you can eat whatever you want.

Alternate day modified fasting (ADMF): Restricting calories to eat no more than a quarter of your recommended baseline energy needs on fasting days, then eating what you want on the alternating days.

Alternative medicine: Practices not generally recognized by the medical community as standard or conventional medical approaches.

Alzheimer's disease: A disease in which nerve cells in the brain degenerate, the brain shrinks, and cognition and memory behavior are impaired.

Anabolic, Anabolism: The processes of the metabolism that generate growth.

Adenosine triphosphate (ATP): a molecule that transfers energy into cells.

Autophagy: A metabolic process triggered by fasting in which a cell rids itself of old, damaged, or abnormal parts.

Bulletproof coffee: A type of coffee with added fat (like grass-fed butter, coconut oil, or MCT oil).

Calorie: How much energy is released when the body breaks down food.

Calorie restriction (CR): Limiting the amount of food you consume while still meeting essential nutritional needs. It is measured by the number of calories eaten in a day.

Cancer: A term that encompasses more than 100 diseases in which cells grow abnormally fast.

Carbohydrate: One of the four basic biomolecules that include sugars, starches, cellulose, and gums that the body converts into the nutrient glucose.

Catabolic, Catabolism: The processes of the metabolism that generate energy.

Chemotherapy: Toxic drugs that are used to kill cancerous cells.

Cholesterol: A type of fat that circulates in your blood. It comes from animal-based food and can also be made in the body.

Circadian rhythm: The internal 24-hour cycle that regulates our bodies, minds and emotions.

Clinical trial: A research program that involves human subjects, used to evaluate various treatments, drugs, or devices.

Diabetes: A dysregulation of blood sugar in the body. Diabetes is caused when the body produces too little insulin or cannot use it properly.

Electrolytes: Minerals that conduct electrical signals throughout the body for nerve and muscle function and help regulate the balance of bodily fluids.

Fat: The most concentrated source of energy for the body. An essential part of our diet, along with protein and carbohydrates.

Food addiction (FA): Excessive consumption of highly palatable foods (i.e., foods high in salt, fat, and sugar) in quantities beyond homeostatic energy requirements.

Glucagon: Hormone released by the pancreas that triggers glycogen molecules to release glucose.

Glucose: Sugar that is released in the blood during digestion and can be stored in the form of fat.

Glycogen: A molecule that stores glucose in the liver.

Homeostasis: The process by which the body coordinates the trillions of cells, 78 organs, and 10 body systems that keep us alive.

Intermittent fasting (IF): An eating plan that restricts when you eat rather than how much you eat. There are many forms of IF.

Ketone, Ketone bodies: An alternate fuel source created when your body burns fat instead of glucose for energy. Ketones also generate more energy than glucose, with fewer toxic by-products like free radicals.

Ketosis: A metabolic state in which the body does not have enough glucose to provide energy and starts to use energy stored as fat. The body also starts to make a substance called ketone (which causes side effects such as bad breath on extreme carbohydrate-restricted diets).

Macronutrients: Nutrients that your body needs in relatively large amounts: carbohydrates, proteins, and fats.

Menopause: End of a woman's reproductive years. At this time, menstruation has stopped. Menopause occurs when a woman has not had a menstrual period for a full year.

Metabolism: The process in which your body turns what you consume into energy to handle the bodily functions that keep you alive.

Micronutrients: Nutrients that your body needs in relatively small amounts: vitamins and minerals.

Perimenopause: The time of a woman's life when menstrual periods become irregular. Refers to the time leading up to menopause.

Periodic fasting (PF): Fasting one or two days a week and eating whatever you want on the other days.

Saturated fat: Fat that is found in red meat, dairy products, and tropical oils. Your body needs a limited amount of saturated fat.

Time-restricted eating, also called time-restricted feeding (TRF): Only eating food during certain hours of the day.

Trans fat: Found in fried and processed foods and made from hydrogenated oil; trans fat is very bad for you.

Unsaturated fat: Fats found in plants and are liquid at room temperature. Your body needs these fats for your brain, metabolism, and blood sugar.

References

8+ Workout log examples. (n.d.). www.examples.com. https://www.examples.com/education/workout-log.html

Adelayanti, N. (2020, April 23). *Fasting as a way to boost your immune system.* www.ugm.ac.id. https://www.ugm.ac.id/en/news/19336-fasting-as-a-way-to-boost-your-immune-system

Aging changes in immunity. (n.d.). Medlineplus.gov. https://medlineplus.gov/ency/article/004008.htm#:~:text=As%20you%20grow%20older%2C%20your

Aging changes in the female reproductive system. (n.d.). Medlineplus.gov. https://medlineplus.gov/ency/article/004016.htm#:~:text=Increased%20risk%20for%20bone%20loss

Agoulnik, D., Lalonde, M. P., Ellmore, G. S., & McKeown, N. M. (2021). Part 1: The Origin and Evolution of the Paleo Diet. *Nutrition Today, 56*(3), 94–104. https://doi.org/10.1097/NT.0000000000000482

Akram, M. (2020, October 18). *HIIT And Intermittent Fasting: Pros, Cons & Workout.* The Fitness Phantom. https://thefitnessphantom.com/hiit-and-intermittent-fasting

Aksungar, F. B., Topkaya, A. E., & Akyildiz, M. (2007). Interleukin-6, C-reactive protein and biochemical parameters during prolonged intermittent fasting. *Annals of Nutrition & Metabolism, 51*(1), 88–95. https://doi.org/10.1159/000100954

Alan Cott. (n.d.). International Society for Orthomolecular Medicine. https://isom.ca/profile/alan-cott/

Amir Adhamy. (2019). *What cells in the human body live the longest?* BBC Science Focus Magazine; https://www.sciencefocus.com/the-human-body/what-cells-in-the-human-body-live-the-longest/

Anderson, M. (2021, August 3). *Intermittent fasting may give your immune system a boost.* Shape. https://www.shape.com/lifestyle/mind-and-body/intermittent-fasting-immune-system

Andrew Rader Studios. (2018). *Cell structure: mitochondria.* Biology4kids.com. http://www.biology4kids.com/files/cell_mito.html

Anton, S. D., Moehl, K., Donahoo, W. T., Marosi, K., Lee, S. A., Mainous, A. G., Leeuwenburgh, C., & Mattson, M. P. (2018). Flipping the metabolic switch: understanding and applying the health benefits of fasting. *Obesity, 26*(2), 254–268. https://doi.org/10.1002/oby.22065

Aurametrix. (2009, December 12). *Vinegar and water diet.* Health Technologies. https://aurametrix.blogspot.com/2009/12/vinegar-and-water-diet.html

Autophagy: your body's natural mechanism to fat burning. (2017, May 5). Simply Health. https://simplyhealthandweightloss.com/blog/autophagy-your-bodys-natural-mechanism-to-fat-burning/

Bagherniya, M., Butler, A. E., Barreto, G. E., & Sahebkar, A. (2018). The effect of fasting or calorie restriction on autophagy induction: A review of the literature. *Ageing Research Reviews, 47,* 183–197. https://doi.org/10.1016/j.arr.2018.08.004

Bathina, S., & Das, U. N. (2015). Brain-derived neurotrophic factor and its clinical implications. *Archives of Medical Science, 6,* 1164–1178. https://doi.org/10.5114/aoms.2015.56342

Bekman, S. (n.d.). *Introduction to fasting.* Stason.org. https://stason.org/TULARC/health/alternative-medicine/Introduction-to-Fasting.html

Benton, E. (2019, December 8). *Attention, attention: keto and low-carb diets are not the same thing.* Women's Health. https://www.womenshealthmag.com/weight-loss/a29833780/low-carb-vs-keto-diet/?utm_source=google&utm_medium=cpc&utm_campaign=arb_ga_whm_md_pmx_us_urlx&gclid=Cj0KCQjwyOuYBh CGARIsAIdGQRMNcB2hA58pm71z63WWDXSvb5UTOjaE iPxPXeDBooZqlmaB9iWfDNIaAnxtEALw_wcB

Berthelot, E., Etchecopar-Etchart, D., Thellier, D., Lancon, C., Boyer, L., & Fond, G. (2021). Fasting interventions for stress, anxiety and depressive symptoms: a systematic review and meta-analysis. *Nutrients, 13*(11), 3947. https://doi.org/10.3390/nu13113947

Bilsborough, S. A., & Crowe, T. C. (2003). Low-carbohydrate diets: what are the potential short- and long-term health implications? *Asia Pacific Journal of Clinical Nutrition, 12*(4), 396–404. https://pubmed.ncbi.nlm.nih.gov/14672862/#:~:text=Compli cations%20such%20as%20heart%20arrhythmias

Björkholm, C., & Monteggia, L. M. (2016). BDNF – a key transducer of antidepressant effects. *Neuropharmacology, 102*, 72–79. https://doi.org/10.1016/j.neuropharm.2015.10.034

Books by David Ortner (author of The 5). (n.d.). www.goodreads.com. https://www.goodreads.com/author/list/8319430.David_Ort ner

Boynton, E. (2022, January 19). *What causes weight gain during menopause?* Right as Rain by UW Medicine. https://rightasrain.uwmedicine.org/well/health/menopause-weight-gain#:~:text=On%20average%2C%20women%20gain%205

Brazier, Y. (2019, February 18). *South beach diet: phases, benefits, what can i eat?* www.medicalnewstoday.com. https://www.medicalnewstoday.com/articles/7501#_noHeaderPrefixedContent

Brill, J. B. (n.d.). *Intermittent fasting and the Mediterranean dDiet - a match made in health heaven.* ModifyHealth. https://modifyhealth.com/blogs/blog/intermittent-fasting-and-the-mediterranean-diet-a-match-made-in-health-heaven

Bulletproof Staff. (2020, October 28). *Can you take supplements while fasting? What you need to know.* Bulletproof. https://www.bulletproof.com/supplements/dietary-supplements/supplements-while-fasting/

Byakodi, R. (2021, November 16). *Intermittent fasting and HIIT: should you combine the two?* 21 Day Hero. https://21dayhero.com/intermittent-fasting-hiit/

BYJUS Staff. (2017, November 21). *Lysosomes.* BYJUS. https://byjus.com/biology/lysosomes/

CAI Editor. (2018, July 27). *Fasting around the world.* Cultural Awareness. https://culturalawareness.com/fasting-around-the-world/

Calorie restriction and fasting diets: What do we know? (2018, August 14). National Institute on Aging. https://www.nia.nih.gov/news/calorie-restriction-and-fasting-diets-what-do-we-know

Can genes be turned on and off in cells? MedlinePlus Genetics. (2021, March 26). Medlineplus.gov. https://medlineplus.gov/genetics/understanding/howgeneswork/geneonoff/#:~:text=Genes%20are%20turned%20on%20and

Can intermittent fasting really improve my gut health? (2021, July 15). Dr. Maura. https://drmaura.com/can-intermittent-fasting-really-improve-my-gut-health/

Cancer and fasting. (2014). UCSF Osher Center for Integrative Medicine. https://osher.ucsf.edu/patient-care/integrative-medicine-resources/cancer-and-nutrition/faq/cancer-and-fasting-calorie-restriction

Carbohydrates. (2012, September 18). The Nutrition Source; Harvard T. H. Chan School of Public Health. https://www.hsph.harvard.edu/nutritionsource/carbohydrates/#:~:text=But%20carbohydrate%20quality%20is%20important

Cardoza, R. (2020, December 11). *22 Easy ways to cut back on carbs.* Eat This Not That. https://www.eatthis.com/reduce-carb-intake/

Caron, J. P., Kreher, M. A., Mickle, A. M., Wu, S., Przkora, R., Estores, I. M., & Sibille, K. T. (2022). Intermittent fasting: potential utility in the treatment of chronic pain across the clinical spectrum. *Nutrients,* *14*(12), 2536. https://doi.org/10.3390/nu14122536

Carroll, C. (2022, June 30). *What is Weight Watchers?* Verywell Fit. https://www.verywellfit.com/weight-watchers-overview-4691074

Cedars-Sinai Staff. (2019, April 16). *Autophagy: recycling is good for your body too.* Cedars-Sinai. https://www.cedars-sinai.org/blog/autophagy.html

Cellante, L. (2020, September 22). *PCOS Facts and myths and how intermittent fasting can help.* LIFE Apps. https://lifeapps.io/fasting/pcos-facts-and-myths-and-how-intermittent-fasting-can-help/

Chandler, B. (2019, July 5). *How to fast one day a week for weight loss.* livestrong.com. https://www.livestrong.com/article/335557-how-to-fast-one-day-a-week-for-weight-loss/

Cherney, K. (2019, February 5). *Effects of menopause on the body.* Healthline.

https://www.healthline.com/health/menopause/hrt-effects-on-body

Cho, D. J. (2020, January 22). *Stars Who've found success with intermittent fasting.* People Magazine. https://people.com/health/stars-who-do-intermittent-fasting/#:~:text=Jennifer%20Aniston&text=%22I%20do%20intermittent%20fasting%2C%20so

Cienfuegos, S., Corapi, S., Gabel, K., Ezpeleta, M., Kalam, F., Lin, S., Pavlou, V., & Varady, K. A. (2022). Effect of intermittent fasting on reproductive hormone levels in females and males: a review of human trials. *Nutrients, 14*(11), 2343. https://doi.org/10.3390/nu14112343

Cleveland Clinic Staff. (n.d.-a). *Perimenopause: age, stages, signs, symptoms & treatment.* Cleveland Clinic. https://my.clevelandclinic.org/health/diseases/21608-perimenopause

Cleveland Clinic Staff. (n.d.-b). *Serotonin: what is it, function & levels.* Cleveland Clinic. https://my.clevelandclinic.org/health/articles/22572-serotonin#:~:text=When%20serotonin%20is%20at%20normal

Cleveland Clinic Staff. (2020, June 5). *Quick, easy ways to get good fats into your diet.* Health Essentials from Cleveland Clinic. https://health.clevelandclinic.org/5-tips-for-eating-good-fats/

Cleveland Clinic Staff. (2021a, January 5). *What is the atkins diet, and is it healthy?* Cleveland Clinic. https://health.clevelandclinic.org/what-is-the-atkins-diet-and-is-it-healthy/#:~:text=Cardiologist%20Robert%20Atkins%20created%20the

Cleveland Clinic Staff. (2021b, March 4). *Why are certain foods so addictive?* Health Essentials from Cleveland Clinic.

https://health.clevelandclinic.org/why-are-certain-foods-so-addictive/

Cleveland Clinic Staff. (2021c, April 15). *Fasting, health & immunity: is there a connection?* Cleveland Clinic Abu Dhabi. https://www.clevelandclinicabudhabi.ae/en/health-byte/pages/fasting-health-immunity-is-there-a-connection.aspx#:~:text=Fasting%20and%20immunity

Cleveland Clinic Staff. (2021d, July 13). *Catabolism vs. anabolism: what's the difference?* Cleveland Clinic. https://health.clevelandclinic.org/anabolism-vs-catabolism/

Cleveland Clinic Staff. (2021e, July 28). *Inflammation: what is it, causes, symptoms & treatment.* Cleveland Clinic. https://my.clevelandclinic.org/health/symptoms/21660-inflammation

Cleveland Clinic Staff. (2021f, October 5). *Menopause: age, stages, signs, symptoms & treatment.* Cleveland Clinic. https://my.clevelandclinic.org/health/diseases/21841-menopause

Cleveland Clinic Staff. (2021g, October 24). *Androgens: function, measurement and related disorders.* Cleveland Clinic. https://my.clevelandclinic.org/health/articles/22002-androgens

Cleveland Clinic Staff. (2022, March 23). *Is it bad to eat before bed?* Cleveland Clinic. https://health.clevelandclinic.org/is-eating-before-bed-bad-for-you/#:~:text=No%2C%20you%20shouldn

Colette. (2022, April 22). The facts behind intermittent fasting with keto diet: benefits, rules, and the atkins approach. Atkins. https://www.atkins.com/how-it-works/blog/the-facts-behind-intermittent-fasting

Collier, R. (2013). Intermittent fasting: the science of going without. *Canadian Medical Association Journal, 185*(9), E363–E364. https://doi.org/10.1503/cmaj.109-4451

Collins, A. (2020, February 21). *Ask Dr Adam | which is best to skip, breakfast, lunch or dinner?* https://formnutrition.com/us/inform/best-meal-to-skip/

Life span of human cells defined: most cells are younger than the individual. (2005, August 12). CORDIS. https://cordis.europa.eu/article/id/24286-life-span-of-human-cells-defined-most-cells-are-younger-than-the-individual

Cronkleton, E. (2017). *What happens if you eat too much protein?* Healthline. https://www.healthline.com/health/too-much-protein

Cross, M. (2021, June 1). *How intermittent fasting can benefit your mental health.* Nutritionist-Resource. https://www.nutritionist-resource.org.uk/memberarticles/how-intermittent-fasting-can-benefit-your-mental-health#:~:text=Yes%2C%20according%20to%20the%20research

Dai, S., Wei, J., Zhang, H., Luo, P., Yang, Y., Jiang, X., Fei, Z., Liang, W., Jiang, J., & Li, X. (2022). Intermittent fasting reduces neuroinflammation in intracerebral hemorrhage through the Sirt3/Nrf2/HO-1 pathway. *Journal of Neuroinflammation, 19*(1), 122. https://doi.org/10.1186/s12974-022-02474-2

Davidson, K. (2020, December 3). *5 Tips for developing a better relationship with food.* Healthline. https://www.healthline.com/nutrition/fixing-a-bad-relationship-with-food#understanding

Davis, C. P. (2021, March 22). *How long do you need to fast for autophagy?* MedicineNet. https://www.medicinenet.com/how_long_do_you_need_to_fast_for_autophagy/article.htm

Delay, don't deny: living an intermittent fasting lifestyle: Stephens, Gin, (2022). Amazon. https://www.amazon.com/Delay-Dont-Deny-Intermittent-Lifestyle/dp/1541325842#:~:text=Gin%20Stephens%20is%20the%20author

Diet review: intermittent fasting for weight loss. (2018, January 16). The Nutrition Source; Harvard T. H. Chan School of Public Health. https://www.hsph.harvard.edu/nutritionsource/healthy-weight/diet-reviews/intermittent-fasting/#:~:text=A%20systematic%20review%20of%2040

DiGiacinto, J., & Spritzler, F. (2016, June 13). *15 Easy ways to reduce your carbohydrate intake.* Healthline. https://www.healthline.com/nutrition/15-ways-to-eat-less-carbs

Djublonskopf. (2015, March 24). *Fletcherism: The hilariously weird fad diet (1903).* Secret History. https://www.djublonskopf.com/2015/03/24/fletcherism-the-hilariously-weird-fad-diet/#:~:text=Horace%20Fletcher%E2%80%94whose%20diet%20earned

Dolson, L. (2016, February 28). *How to calculate your protein needs.* Verywell Fit; https://www.verywellfit.com/how-to-calculate-how-much-protein-you-need-3955709

Dolson, L. (2019). *How to cut carbs: 10 must-have tips.* Verywell Fit. https://www.verywellfit.com/tips-for-cutting-carbs-2242032

Dwivedi, Y. (2009). Brain-derived neurotrophic factor: role in depression and suicide. *Neuropsychiatric Disease and Treatment, 5,* 433–449. https://www.ncbi.nlm.nih.gov/pmc/articles/PMC2732010/

Ellis, S. (2017, March 10). *How should you exercise while you're intermittent fasting? Doctors weigh in.* Mindbodygreen.

https://www.mindbodygreen.com/0-29179/how-should-you-exercise-while-youre-intermittent-fasting-doctors-weigh-in.html

Elson M. Haas. (n.d.). WebMD. https://www.webmd.com/elson-m-haas

Etienne-Mesubi, M. (2021, February 16). *The right way to do OMAD (one meal a day).* LIFE Apps. https://lifeapps.io/fasting/the-right-way-to-do-omad-one-meal-a-day/

Fasting and autophagy. (n.d.). Spartan Medical Associates. https://www.spartanmedicalassociates.com/fasting-and-autophagy/#:~:text=Fasting%20is%20a%20great%20stimulus

Fasting and mitochondrial health. (n.d.). The Institute for Functional Medicine. https://www.ifm.org/news-insights/fasting-mitochondrial-health/

Fasting: ancient wisdom for modern times. (2022, January 5). Holistic Lakewood. https://holisticlakewood.com/fasting-ancient-wisdom-for-modern-times/

Fats and cholesterol. (2012, September 18). The Nutrition Source; Harvard T. H. Chan School of Public Health. https://www.hsph.harvard.edu/nutritionsource/what-should-you-eat/fats-and-cholesterol/#:~:text=Choose%20foods%20with%20

Fit for life diet.. (n.d.). www.encyclopedia.com. https://www.encyclopedia.com/science/encyclopedias-almanacs-transcripts-and-maps/fit-life-diet

Foley, K. E. (2018, September 1). *A short history of terrible diets.* Quartz. https://qz.com/quartzy/1374958/a-short-history-of-terrible-diets/

Food addiction - an overview. (n.d.). Science Direct. https://www.sciencedirect.com/topics/medicine-and-dentistry/food-addiction#:~:text=Abstract-

Fuentes, L. (2021, December 15). *Start easy with the 12-hour intermittent fasting method.* Laura Fuentes. https://www.laurafuentes.com/12-hour-intermittent-fasting/

Fung, J. (2015, April 11). *Fasting – a history part I.* The Fasting Method. https://blog.thefastingmethod.com/fasting-a-history-part-i/#:~:text=Fasting%20is%20a%20time%20tested

Furmli, S., Elmasry, R., Ramos, M., & Fung, J. (2018). Therapeutic use of intermittent fasting for people with type 2 diabetes as an alternative to insulin. *BMJ Case Reports,* bcr-2017-221854. https://doi.org/10.1136/bcr-2017-221854

Gahl, W. (2019). *Mitochondria.* National Human Genome Research Institute. https://www.genome.gov/genetics-glossary/Mitochondria

Geurin, L. (2021, December 23). *42 Intermittent fasting quotes to motivate you.* LoriGeurin.com. https://lorigeurin.com/intermittent-fasting-quotes/

Goldhamer, A., Helms, S., & Salloum, T. K. (2015, June 23). Fasting. https://clinicalgate.com/fasting/

Gotthardt, J. D., Verpeut, J. L., Yeomans, B. L., Yang, J. A., Yasrebi, A., Roepke, T. A., & Bello, N. T. (2016). Intermittent fasting promotes fat loss with lean mass retention, increased hypothalamic norepinephrine content, and increased neuropeptide y gene expression in diet-induced obese male mice. *Endocrinology, 157*(2), 679–691. https://doi.org/10.1210/en.2015-1622

Griffith, T. (2017, October 16). *Fasting and cancer.* Healthline. https://www.healthline.com/health/fasting-and-cancer

Gudden, J., Arias Vasquez, A., & Bloemendaal, M. (2021). The effects of intermittent fasting on brain and cognitive function. *Nutrients, 13*(9), 3166. https://doi.org/10.3390/nu13093166

Gunnars, K. (2016, August 16). *10 Evidence-based health benefits of intermittent fasting*. Healthline. https://www.healthline.com/nutrition/10-health-benefits-of-intermittent-fasting

Gunnars, K. (2017). *10 High-fat foods that are actually super healthy*. Healthline. https://www.healthline.com/nutrition/10-super-healthy-high-fat-foods

Haas, E. M. (n.d.). *Nutritional program for fasting - Elson M. Haas M.D.* Hawsedc. Retrieved August 29, 2022, from http://hawsedc.com/tom/haasfasting.htm

Hannan, A., Rahman, A., Rahman, S., Sohag, A. A. M., Dash, R., Hossain, K. S., Farjana, M., & Uddin, J. (2020). Intermittent fasting, a possible priming tool for host defense against SARS-CoV-2 infection: Crosstalk among calorie restriction, autophagy and immune response. *Immunology Letters, 226*, 38–45. https://doi.org/10.1016/j.imlet.2020.07.001

Harris, S. (2020, January 5). *What happens if you don't eat for a day? Timeline and effects*. Medical NewsToday. https://www.medicalnewstoday.com/articles/322065#:~:text=As%20well%20as%20aiding%20weight

Harvard School of Public Health. (2015, April 8). *Healthy eating plate vs. USDA's MyPlate*. The Nutrition Source. https://www.hsph.harvard.edu/nutritionsource/healthy-eating-plate-vs-usda-myplate/

Healthwise Staff. (2021, July 28). *Carbohydrates, proteins, fats, and blood sugar*. Myhealth. https://myhealth.alberta.ca/Health/Pages/conditions.aspx?hwid=uq1238abc#:~:text=Carbohydrates%20are%20used%20for%20energy

Hensley, S. (2011, December 6). Feds say HCG diet remedies are "illegal." *NPR*. https://www.npr.org/sections/health-shots/2011/12/06/143212937/feds-say-hcg-diet-remedies-are-illegal

High-protein diets -- do they really work? (2019). Nourish by WebMD; WebMD. https://www.webmd.com/diet/ss/slideshow-high-protein-diet

Hill, A. (2020, January 7). *Eat stop eat review: does it work for weight loss?* Healthline. https://www.healthline.com/nutrition/eat-stop-eat-review#effectiveness

History of therapeutic fasting. (n.d.). Buchinger Wilhelmi. https://www.buchinger-wilhelmi.com/en/geschichte-des-heilfastens/

Hodapp, P. (n.d.). *Intermittent fasting + mitochondria (why you should care).* Spartan Race. https://www.spartan.com/blogs/unbreakable-nutrition/intermittent-fasting-mitochondria#:~:text=Intermittent%20fasting%20focuses%20on%20%5Bmitochondria

Homberg, J. R., Molteni, R., Calabrese, F., & Riva, M. A. (2014). The serotonin–BDNF duo: Developmental implications for the vulnerability to psychopathology. *Neuroscience & Biobehavioral Reviews, 43,* 35–47. https://doi.org/10.1016/j.neubiorev.2014.03.012

Hormonal Weight Gain. (2022). Endocrinology Consultants, P.C. https://www.endocrinewellness.com/hormonal-weight-gain/

Horne, B. D., Muhlestein, J. B., & Anderson, J. L. (2015). Health effects of intermittent fasting: hormesis or harm? A systematic review. *The American Journal of Clinical Nutrition, 102*(2), 464–470. https://doi.org/10.3945/ajcn.115.109553

Intermittent fasting and high intensity interval training. (2020, December 28). Bob Gardner Fitness & Nutrition. https://bobgardnerfitness.com/intermittent-fasting-high-intensity-interval-training/

Intermittent fasting may be center of increasing lifespan. (2017, November 3). Harvard Gazette. https://news.harvard.edu/gazette/story/2017/11/intermittent-fasting-may-be-center-of-increasing-lifespan/

Intermountain Healthcare. (2022, July 7). *Study finds people who practice intermittent fasting experience less severe complications from COVID-19.* EurekAlert! https://www.eurekalert.org/news-releases/958151

Jarreau, P. (2021, June 1). *The 5 stages of intermittent fasting.* LIFE Apps. https://lifeapps.io/fasting/the-5-stages-of-intermittent-fasting/#:~:text=The%205%20Stages%20of%20Intermittent%20Fasting%20with%20the%20LIFE%20Fasting

Jason Fung, MD. (n.d.). The Institute for Functional Medicine. https://www.ifm.org/about/profile/jason-fung-md/#:~:text=Jason%20Fung%2C%20MD%2C%20was%20born

Jess. (2013, July 17). *17 Benefits of eating paleo.* Paleo Grubs; https://paleogrubs.com/paleo-benefits

Johns Hopkins Medicine Staff. (2020). *Introduction to menopause.* Johns Hopkins Medicine. https://www.hopkinsmedicine.org/health/conditions-and-diseases/introduction-to-menopause

Johnson, J. B., Laub, D. R., & John, S. (2006). The effect on health of alternate day calorie restriction: Eating less and more than needed on alternate days prolongs life. *Medical Hypotheses, 67*(2), 209–211. https://doi.org/10.1016/j.mehy.2006.01.030

Johnson, J. B., Summer, W., Cutler, R. G., Martin, B., Hyun, D.-H., Dixit, V. D., Pearson, M., Nassar, M., Tellejohan, R., Maudsley, S., Carlson, O., John, S., Laub, D. R., & Mattson, M. P. (2007). Alternate day calorie restriction improves clinical findings and reduces markers of oxidative stress and inflammation in overweight adults with moderate asthma. *Free Radical Biology and*

Medicine, *42*(5), 665–674. https://doi.org/10.1016/j.freeradbiomed.2006.12.005

Just Skip A Meal. (2022). Metabolic Research Center. https://www.emetabolic.com/locations/centers/cary/blog/we ight-loss/spontaneous-meal-skipping-is-an-informal-fasting-protocol/#:~:text=Intermittent%20fasting%20is%20simply%2 0a

Kandola, A. (2019a, January 2). *7 filling foods to prevent hunger backed by science.* Medical News Today. https://www.medicalnewstoday.com/articles/324078

Kandola, A. (2019b, May 14). *Simple carbs vs. complex carbs: What's the difference?* Medical News Today. https://www.medicalnewstoday.com/articles/325171

Kättström, D. (2019, December 23). *The ancient phenomenon of fasting.* Food Pharmacy. https://foodpharmacyco.com/2019/12/the-ancient-phenomenon-of-fasting/

Kaupe, A. (2019, March 8). *How to do intermittent fasting according to 40 famous people.* 21 Day Hero. https://21dayhero.com/how-to-do-intermittent-fasting-according-to-famous-people/

Kelli. (2022, January 3). *Printable intermittent fasting schedule.* Freebie Finding Mom. https://www.freebiefindingmom.com/printable-intermittent-fasting-schedule/

Ketones vs. glucose - interesting facts. (2021, December 11). Bio Chem. https://bio-chem.co.il/en/articles-en/ketones-vs-glucose-interesting-facts/

Klimars, E. (2019, March 27). *This is what intermittent fasting does to your brain.* Radboud Universiteit. https://www.ru.nl/@1211513/what-intermittent-fasting-does-your-brain/#:~:text=After%20only%20about%20six%20hours

Kubala, J. (2018a, July 3). *The warrior diet: review and beginner's guide.* Healthline. https://www.healthline.com/nutrition/warrior-diet-guide

Kubala, J. (2018b, November 5). *Intermittent fasting and keto: Should you combine the two?* Healthline. https://www.healthline.com/nutrition/intermittent-fasting-and-keto

Kubala, J. (2020, January 7). *Why is the keto diet good for you?* Medical News Today. https://www.medicalnewstoday.com/articles/319196

Landau, M. D. (2022, January 19). *Intermittent fasting around menopause: Does it make sense?* EverydayHealth.com. https://www.everydayhealth.com/womens-health/what-midlife-women-should-know-about-intermittent-fasting/

Leonard, J. (2020, January 17). *16:8 intermittent fasting: Benefits, how-to, and tips.* Medical News Today. https://www.medicalnewstoday.com/articles/327398

Lett, R. (2021, September 8). *Guide to managing hunger, while intermittent fasting.* Span Health. https://www.span.health/blog/guide-to-hunger-while-intermittent-fasting

Licalzi, D. (2021, June 28). *Autophagy: what you should know before starting your fast.* Blog.insidetracker.com. https://blog.insidetracker.com/autophagy-know-before-starting-fast

Lindberg, S. (2018, August 23). *Autophagy: definition, diet, fasting, cancer, benefits, and more.* Healthline. https://www.healthline.com/health/autophagy

Lindberg, S. (2020, September 1). *How to exercise safely during intermittent fasting.* Healthline. https://www.healthline.com/health/how-to-exercise-safely-intermittent-fasting

Link, R. (2018a, July 30). *8 Health benefits of fasting, backed by science.* Healthline. https://www.healthline.com/nutrition/fasting-benefits#TOC_TITLE_HDR_2

Link, R. (2018b, September 4). *16/8 Intermittent fasting: a beginner's guide.* Healthline; Healthline Media. https://www.healthline.com/nutrition/16-8-intermittent-fasting

London, I. C. (2022, July 3). *Nerve regeneration and repair: Intermittent fasting may help heal nerve damage.* SciTechDaily. https://scitechdaily.com/nerve-regeneration-and-repair-intermittent-fasting-may-help-heal-nerve-damage/#:~:text=Nerve%20Regeneration%20and%20Repair%3A%20Intermittent%20Fasting%20May%20Help%20Heal%20Nerve%20Damage

Long-haul COVID deserves more attention, UTSW expert says. (2022, August 23). www.utsouthwestern.edu. https://www.utsouthwestern.edu/newsroom/articles/year-2022/august-long-haul-covid.html

Longo, V. D., & Cortellino, S. (2020). Fasting, dietary restriction, and immunosenescence. *Journal of Allergy and Clinical Immunology, 146*(5), 1002–1004. https://doi.org/10.1016/j.jaci.2020.07.035

Longo, Valter D., & Mattson, Mark P. (2014). fasting: molecular mechanisms and clinical applications. *Cell Metabolism, 19*(2), 181–192. https://doi.org/10.1016/j.cmet.2013.12.008

Low-fat diets for weight loss. (2002, April 12). WebMD. https://www.webmd.com/women/reducing-dietary-fat

Magee, E. (2005, February 18). *Your "Hunger Hormones.* WebMD. https://www.webmd.com/diet/features/your-hunger-hormones

Marcin, A. (2017, September 18). *What's the average weight for women?* Healthline. https://www.healthline.com/health/womens-health/average-weight-for-women

Mawer, R. (2019, September 23). *11 Ways to boost human growth hormone (HGH) naturally.* Healthline. https://www.healthline.com/nutrition/11-ways-to-increase-hgh

Mayer, K. (2021, September 29). *Intermittent fasting extends healthspan through circadian autophagy.* Genetic Engineering and Biotechnology News. https://www.genengnews.com/news/intermittent-fasting-extends-healthspan-through-circadian-autophagy/

Mayo Clinic Staff. (n.d.). *Can a low-carb diet help you lose weight?* Mayo Clinic. https://www.mayoclinic.org/healthy-lifestyle/weight-loss/in-depth/low-carb-diet/art-20045831#:~:text=Insulin%20is%20released%20to%20help

Mayo Clinic Staff. (2017). *South Beach Diet.* Mayo Clinic. https://www.mayoclinic.org/healthy-lifestyle/weight-loss/in-depth/south-beach-diet/art-20048491

Mayo Clinic Staff. (2019). *Perimenopause - Symptoms and causes.* Mayo Clinic. https://www.mayoclinic.org/diseases-conditions/perimenopause/symptoms-causes/syc-20354666

Mayo Clinic Staff. (2019, June 8). *Frequently asked questions about stem cell research.* Mayo Clinic. https://www.mayoclinic.org/tests-procedures/bone-marrow-transplant/in-depth/stem-cells/art-20048117#:~:text=Stem%20cell%20therapy%2C%20also%20known

Mayo Clinic Staff. (2020a, September 29). *Can triglycerides affect my heart health?* Mayo Clinic. https://www.mayoclinic.org/diseases-conditions/high-blood-cholesterol/in-depth/triglycerides/art-20048186

Mayo Clinic Staff. (2020b, November 19). *Aging: What to expect*. Mayo Clinic. https://www.mayoclinic.org/healthy-lifestyle/healthy-aging/in-depth/aging/art-20046070#:~:text=Your%20bones%2C%20joints%20and%20muscles&text=With%20age%2C%20bones%20tend%20to

Mayo Clinic Staff. (2022, August 4). *Counting calories: Get back to weight-loss basics*. Mayo Clinic. https://www.mayoclinic.org/healthy-lifestyle/weight-loss/in-depth/calories/art-20048065#:~:text=And%20if%20you%20eat%20fewer

McAllister, E. J., Dhurandhar, N. V., Keith, S. W., Aronne, L. J., Barger, J., Baskin, M., Benca, R. M., Biggio, J., Boggiano, M. M., Eisenmann, J. C., Elobeid, M., Fontaine, K. R., Gluckman, P., Hanlon, E. C., Katzmarzyk, P., Pietrobelli, A., Redden, D. T., Ruden, D. M., Wang, C., & Waterland, R. A. (2009). Ten Putative Contributors to the Obesity Epidemic. *Critical Reviews in Food Science and Nutrition, 49*(10), 868–913. https://doi.org/10.1080/10408390903372599

McGivern, R. (2014). *Chapter 15. Religion – introduction to sociology – 1st Canadian eEdition*. opentextbc.ca. https://opentextbc.ca/introductiontosociology/chapter/chapter-15-religion/

Meixner, M. (2018, October 8). *13 Low-fat foods that are good for your health*. Healthline. https://www.healthline.com/nutrition/healthy-low-fat-foods

Melville, K. (2020, May 14). *Paleo intermittent fasting: how to get the benefits of both diets*. Chris Kresser. https://chriskresser.com/paleo-intermittent-fasting-how-to-get-the-benefits-of-both-diets/

Metabolism overview: anabolism and catabolism (video). (n.d.). Khan Academy. https://www.khanacademy.org/test-prep/mcat/biomolecules/overview-metabolism/v/overview-of-metabolism-anabolism-and-catabolism

Midland, N. (2020, October 8). *2-Day fast for weight loss: a simple metabolism-boosting technique.* BetterMe Blog. https://betterme.world/articles/2-day-fast-weight-loss/

Migala, J. (2019, January 29). *Intermittent fasting keto: how it works, benefits, risks, more..* EverydayHealth. https://www.everydayhealth.com/ketogenic-diet/intermittent-fasting-keto-how-it-works-benefits-risks-more/

Migala, J. (2021, November 18). *OMAD Diet: safety, health benefits, risks, and more.* EverydayHealth. https://www.everydayhealth.com/diet-nutrition/omad-diet/

Miller, K. (2021, March 1). *The eat stop eat diet involves fasting for 24 hours at a time.* Women's Health. https://www.womenshealthmag.com/weight-loss/a22689488/eat-stop-eat-diet/

Miller, S. (2022, May 27). *Intermittent fasting and insulin resistance: benefits beyond weight loss.* www.jeffersonhealth.org. https://www.jeffersonhealth.org/your-health/living-well/intermittent-fasting-and-insulin-resistance-benefits-beyond-weight-loss

Mount Sinai researchers discover that fasting reduces inflammation and improves chronic inflammatory diseases. (2019, August 22). Mount Sinai Health System. https://www.mountsinai.org/about/newsroom/2019/mount-sinai-researchers-discover-that-fasting-reduces-inflammation-and-improves-chronic-inflammatory-diseases#:~:text=Merad%20and%20colleagues%20showed%20that

Mullens, A. (2018, February 4). *Dr. Jason Fung: dismantling diet dogma.* Diet Doctor. https://www.dietdoctor.com/dr-jason-fung-dismantling-diet-dogma-one-puzzle-piece-time

Mulrooney, L. (2022, July 15). *Study: intermittent fasting associated with less severe COVID-19 complications.* Pharmacy Times.

https://www.pharmacytimes.com/view/study-intermittent-fasting-associated-with-less-severe-covid-19-complications

NCI. (n.d.). *Review: introduction to the human body.* training.seer.cancer.gov. https://training.seer.cancer.gov/anatomy/body/review.html#:~:text=A%20system%20is%20an%20organization

Newcomb, B. (2017, March 30). *Fasting during chemotherapy may offset some side effects of cancer-fighting drugs.* USC News. https://news.usc.edu/118758/fasting-during-chemotherapy-may-offset-spikes-in-blood-sugar-caused-by-cancer-fighting-drugs/

NIH Staff. (2017, December). *Your digestive system & how it works.* National Institute of Diabetes and Digestive and Kidney Diseases. https://www.niddk.nih.gov/health-information/digestive-diseases/digestive-system-how-it-works#:~:text=Glands%20in%20your%20stomach%20lining

Parity, M. (2021, May 19). *What to eat if you're intermittent fasting.* The Paleo Diet®. https://thepaleodiet.com/what-to-eat-if-youre-intermittent-fasting

Parker, K. (2021, June 2). *The effect of intermittent fasting on your brain.* Aviv Clinics USA. https://aviv-clinics.com/blog/nutrition/the-effect-of-intermittent-fasting-on-your-brain/#:~:text=Intermittent%20fasting%20is%20amazing%20for

Peeke, P. (2010, April 20). *Eating when you're tired.* WebMD. https://blogs.webmd.com/from-our-archives/20100420/eating-when-youre-tired#:~:text=The%20stomach%20secretes%20the%20hormone

Piersol, B. (2020, October 9). *Intermittent fasting and breast cancer: what you need to know.* Memorial Sloan Kettering Cancer Center. https://www.mskcc.org/news/intermittent-fasting-and-breast-cancer-what-you-need-know

Poff, A. M., Ari, C., Arnold, P., Seyfried, T. N., & D'Agostino, D. P. (2014). Ketone supplementation decreases tumor cell viability and prolongs survival of mice with metastatic cancer. *International Journal of Cancer, 135*(7), 1711–1720. https://doi.org/10.1002/ijc.28809

Poljšak, B., & Milisav, I. (2012). Clinical implications of cellular stress responses. *Bosnian Journal of Basic Medical Sciences, 12*(2), 122. https://doi.org/10.17305/bjbms.2012.2510

Preiato, D. (2019, May 23). *48-Hour fast: how-to, benefits, and downsides.* Healthline. https://www.healthline.com/nutrition/48-hour-fasting

Pritikin Diet. (n.d.). www.encyclopedia.com. https://www.encyclopedia.com/science/encyclopedias-almanacs-transcripts-and-maps/pritikin-diet

Rabinowitz, J. D., & White, E. (2010). Autophagy and metabolism. *Science, 330*(6009), 1344–1348. https://doi.org/10.1126/science.1193497

Raman, R. (2017, April 4). *The zone diet: a complete overview.* Healthline. https://www.healthline.com/nutrition/zone-diet#:~:text=What%20is%20the%20Zone%20Diet

Rana, S. (2018, May 2). *Sleeping beauty diet: the bizarre diet fad people are embracing to lose weight.* NDTV Food. https://food.ndtv.com/food-drinks/sleeping-beauty-diet-the-bizarre-diet-fad-people-are-embracing-to-lose-weight-1733037

Research on intermittent fasting shows health benefits. (2020, February 27). National Institute on Aging. https://www.nia.nih.gov/news/research-intermittent-fasting-shows-health-benefits

Richards, L. (2020, December 21). Everything to know about The Warrior Diet. *Medical News Today.* https://www.medicalnewstoday.com/articles/warrior-diet

Rizzo, N. (2022, January 31). *The best foods for an intermittent fasting diet.* Greatist. https://greatist.com/eat/what-to-eat-on-an-intermittent-fasting-diet#different-methods

Rogers, K. (2019). Biomolecule. *Encyclopædia Britannica.* https://www.britannica.com/science/biomolecule

Rotter, J. (2017, September 15). *11 Things women should know about menopause.* Healthline. https://www.healthline.com/health/menopause/menopause-facts#menopause-age

Salomon, S. H., & Lawler, M. (2022, June 10). *8 Scientific health benefits of the mediterranean diet.* EverydayHealth.com. https://www.everydayhealth.com/mediterranean-diet/scientific-health-benefits-mediterranean-diet/

Samuel, L. (2010, July 18). *003 What ATP is and how it works.* www.youtube.com. https://www.youtube.com/watch?v=xUpuuL24NiQ

Schimmel, A. (2019). Rumi. *Encyclopædia Britannica.* https://www.britannica.com/biography/Rumi

Schulz, N. (2012, December 18). *Agricultural abundance: an american innovation story.* U.S. Chamber of Commerce Foundation. https://www.uschamberfoundation.org/agricultural-abundance-american-innovation-story

SCL Health. (n.d.). *How much protein is simply too much?* www.sclhealth.org. https://www.sclhealth.org/blog/2019/07/how-much-protein-is-simply-too-much/

Seitz, A. (2018). *Good fats vs. bad fats: everything you need to know.* Healthline. https://www.healthline.com/health/heart-disease/good-fats-vs-bad-fats

Sex hormone binding globulin (SHBG). (2021, March 24). testing.com. https://www.testing.com/tests/sex-hormone-binding-globulin-shbg/#:~:text=Sex%20hormone%20binding%20globulin%20(SHBG)%20is%20a%20protein%20produced%20by

Shields, A. (2020, November 5). *What actually happens to your body during a fast, hour by hour.* mindbodygreen. https://www.mindbodygreen.com/articles/what-happens-when-you-fast

SlimFast intermittent fasting complete meal bars. (n.d.). Shop SlimFast. https://shop.slimfast.com/collections/all-products/products/slimfast-intermittent-fasting-meal-bars

Smart, W. (2022, March 16). *How intermittent fasting affects your brain health.* joinzoe.com. https://joinzoe.com/learn/intermittent-fasting-and-brain-health

Snyder, C. (2021, January 4). *Always thinking about food? Here's how to stop (9 steps).* Healthline. https://www.healthline.com/nutrition/how-to-stop-thinking-about-food#why-you-think-about-food

Sogawa, H., & Kubo, C. (2000). Influence of short-term repeated fasting on the longevity of female (NZB×NZW)F1 mice. *Mechanisms of Ageing and Development, 115*(1-2), 61–71. https://doi.org/10.1016/s0047-6374(00)00109-3

Spritzler, F. (2021, May 21). *14 Easy ways to increase your protein intake.* Healthline. https://www.healthline.com/nutrition/14-ways-to-increase-protein-intake

Stanton, B., & O'Neill, T. (2021). *How to choose an intermittent fasting schedule.* Carb Manager. https://www.carbmanager.com/article/yoherxeaaceazayu/how-to-choose-an-intermittent-fasting-schedule/

Stenson, J. (2021, August 12). *What we thought about metabolism may be all wrong, new study suggests.* NBC News. https://www.nbcnews.com/health/health-news/metabolism-adulthood-does-not-slow-commonly-believed-study-finds-n1276650

Stuck, R. (n.d.). *Intermittent fasting and the gut microbiome.* Ixcela. https://ixcela.com/resources/intermittent-fasting-and-the-gut-microbiome.html

Study finds routine periodic fasting is good for your health, and your heart. (2011, April 3). EurekAlert! https://www.eurekalert.org/news-releases/906514#:~:text=HGH%20works%20to%20protect%20lean

Susarla, S. (2021, January 13). *Intermittent fasting can enhance the idmmune system.* Susarla Primary Care. https://susarlapc.com/intermittent-fasting-can-enhance-the-immune-system/

Thakkar, P. (2022, June 17). *Here's everything about the deadly "last chance" diet that actually killed people.* www.mensxp.com. https://www.mensxp.com/health/nutrition/51460-here-rsquo-s-everything-about-the-deadly-last-chance-diet-that-actually-killed-people.html

The 12:12 intermittent fasting diet: Can it really boost weight loss and flatten your tummy? (n.d.). www.timesnownews.com. https://www.timesnownews.com/health/article/intermittent-fasting-for-weight-loss-is-the-12-12-diet-plan-best-for-losing-belly-fat-for-beginners/322873

The Chalkboard Editorial Team. (2021, March 16). *Calorie restriction + intermittent fasting are not the same thing according to Dr. Will Cole.* The Chalkboard. https://thechalkboardmag.com/calorie-restriction-intermittent-fasting

The Editors of Encyclopaedia Britannica. (2019). Fasting. *Encyclopædia Britannica.* https://www.britannica.com/topic/fasting

The emotional roller coaster of menopause. (2021, August 9). WebMD. https://www.webmd.com/menopause/guide/emotional-roller-coaster#:~:text=Irritability%20and%20feelings%20of%20sadness

The joy of fasting. (2020, September 19). The Fasting Flamingo. https://thefastingflamingo.com/the-joy-of-fasting-rumi-poem/

The Live Better Team. (2016, August 22). *How your body systems are connected - revere health.* Revere Health. https://reverehealth.com/live-better/how-body-systems-connected/

The New York Times. (2022, September 6). Coronavirus in the U.S.: latest map and case count. *The New York Times.* https://www.nytimes.com/interactive/2021/us/covid-cases.html

The one addition to the Mediterranean diet that will make it "ideal" for heart health. (2020, September 20). 7NEWS; 7 News. https://7news.com.au/lifestyle/doctors-declare-mediterranean-diet-plus-intermittent-fasting-is-ideal-for-a-healthy-heart--c-1326882

Top 7 quotes by Chris Mohr. (n.d.). A-Z Quotes. https://www.azquotes.com/author/60541-Chris_Mohr

Topness, E. S. (2012). *6 Primary functions of proteins.* Sfgate.com. https://healthyeating.sfgate.com/6-primary-functions-proteins-5372.html

Trafton, A. (2018, May 3). *Fasting boosts stem cells' regenerative capacity.* Massachusetts Institute of Technology. https://news.mit.edu/2018/fasting-boosts-stem-cells-regenerative-capacity-0503

Tramazzo, J. (2019, July 24). *Fasting & autophagy (part 2) — how to trigger & maximize autophagy.* Medium.

https://josephtramazzo.medium.com/autophagy-fasting-part-2-how-to-trigger-maximize-autophagy-78a137b787b7

Trumpfeller, G. (2020a, January 14). *Intermittent fasting and insulin resistance: how the two are connected.* Simple.life Blog. https://simple.life/blog/intermittent-fasting-and-insulin/

Trumpfeller, G. (2020b, January 22). *How much weight can you lose with intermittent fasting?* Simple.life Blog. https://simple.life/blog/intermittent-fasting-weight-loss-results/

Trumpfeller, G. (2020c, April 29). *Does intermittent fasting slow down metabolism? See for yourself.* Simple.life Blog. https://simple.life/blog/intermittent-fasting-and-metabolism/

Trumpfeller, G. (2020d, July 22). *Do you need to take supplements during intermittent fasting?* Simple.life Blog. https://simple.life/blog/intermittent-fasting-and-supplements/

Types of fat. (2014, June 9). The Nutrition Source; Harvard T. H. Chan School of Public Health. https://www.hsph.harvard.edu/nutritionsource/what-should-you-eat/fats-and-cholesterol/types-of-fat/#:~:text=Unsaturated%20fats%2C%20which%20are%20liquid

U.S. News Staff. (2015). *Nutrisystem diet.* usnews.com. https://health.usnews.com/best-diet/nutrisystem-diet

U.S. News Staff. (2019). *Jenny Craig diet.* usnews.com. https://health.usnews.com/best-diet/jenny-craig-diet

UF Health. (2019, February 1). *Flipping the metabolic switch to fight obesity.* UF Health, University of Florida Health. https://ufhealth.org/blog/flipping-metabolic-switch-fight-obesity

Varady, K. A., Bhutani, S., Church, E. C., & Klempel, M. C. (2009). Short-term modified alternate-day fasting: a novel dietary strategy for weight loss and cardioprotection in obese adults. *The American Journal of Clinical Nutrition*, *90*(5), 1138–1143. https://doi.org/10.3945/ajcn.2009.28380

Venus Williams quotes. (n.d.). quotefancy.com. https://quotefancy.com/venus-williams-quotes

Vetter, C. (2022, March 8). *Intermittent fasting, gut health, and your microbiome.* joinzoe.com. https://joinzoe.com/learn/intermittent-fasting-gut-health

Visioli, F., Mucignat-Caretta, C., Anile, F., & Panaite, S.-A. (2022). Traditional and medical applications of fasting. *Nutrients*, *14*(3), 433. https://doi.org/10.3390/nu14030433

Wang, Y., & Wu, R. (2022). The effect of fasting on human metabolism and psychological health. *Disease Markers*, *2022*, 1–7. https://doi.org/10.1155/2022/5653739

Ways to heal your mitochondria: fasting and functional medicine. (2022, May 12). Internal Healing and Wellnessmd. https://internalhealingandwellnessmd.com/a-new-way-to-heal-your-mitochondria-fasting-and-functional-medicine/

WebMD. (2014, September 8). *Ketosis and the keto diet.* WebMD. https://www.webmd.com/diabetes/type-1-diabetes-guide/what-is-ketosis#1

WebMD Editorial Contributors, (n.d.). *Is Eating one meal a day safe?* WebMD. https://www.webmd.com/diet/is-eating-one-meal-a-day-safe

Weight loss programs & plans that work. (n.d.). www.jennycraig.com. https://www.jennycraig.com/how-it-works

Welcome. (n.d.). Valter Longo. https://www.valterlongo.com/#:~:text=Dr.

Welcome to orthomolecular.org. (2017). Orthomolecular.org. http://orthomolecular.org/

Wells, K. (2011, January 8). *Why saturated fat is not the enemy (& why we need It).* Wellness Mama®. https://wellnessmama.com/health/saturated-fat/

West, H. (2021, July 19). *Does intermittent fasting boost your metabolism?* Healthline. https://www.healthline.com/nutrition/intermittent-fasting-metabolism#:~:text=Intermittent%20fasting%20is%20a%20powerful

What is the cellular "metabolic switch" and why is it so important to losing weight? (2020, May 19). Sand Cosmetic. https://www.sandcosmetic.com/blog/what-is-the-cellular-metabolic-switch-and-why-is-it-so-important-to-losing-weight/

What to know about intermittent fasting for women after 50. (2021, September 27). WebMD. https://www.webmd.com/healthy-aging/what-to-know-about-intermittent-fasting-for-women-after-50

Who Is Dr. Elson? (n.d.). Elson Haas, M.D. https://elsonhaasmd.com/who-is-dr-elson/

Wikipedia Contributors. (2019a, June 29). *Whole30.* Wikimedia Foundation. https://en.wikipedia.org/wiki/Whole30

Wikipedia Contributors. (2019b, December 8). *SlimFast.* Wikimedia Foundation. https://en.wikipedia.org/wiki/SlimFast

Wikipedia Contributors. (2020, August 9). *Jenny Craig, Inc.* Wikipedia Foundatton. https://en.wikipedia.org/wiki/Jenny_Craig

Wikipedia Contributors. (2021a, January 27). *Grapefruit diet.* Wikipedia Foundation. https://en.wikipedia.org/wiki/Grapefruit_diet#:~:text=The%20diet%20is%20based%20on

Wikipedia Contributors. (2021b, July 21). *Walter L. Voegtlin*. Wikipedia. Foundation https://en.wikipedia.org/wiki/Walter_L._Voegtlin

Wikipedia Contributors. (2021c, October 2). *Nathan Pritikin*. Wikipedia Foundation. https://en.wikipedia.org/wiki/Nathan_Pritikin

Wikipedia Contributors. (2022, July 27). *Jentezen Franklin*. Wikipedia Foundation. https://en.wikipedia.org/wiki/Jentezen_Franklin

Williams, C. (2018, June 1). *How intermittent fasting affects your metabolism*. Cooking Light. https://www.cookinglight.com/healthy-living/healthy-habits/how-fasting-affects-metabolism

Winterman, D. (2013, January 2). History's weirdest fad diets. *BBC News*. https://www.bbc.com/news/magazine-20695743

Winters, D. (2021, October 15). *How fasting can regenerate immune cells*. Tonic Health. https://www.tonichealth.co/blogs/news/how-fasting-can-regenerate-immune-cells

Wu, S. (2014, June 5). *Fasting triggers stem cell regeneration of damaged, old immune system*. USC News. https://news.usc.edu/63669/fasting-triggers-stem-cell-regeneration-of-damaged-old-immune-system/

Yılmaz, M., & Kayançiçek, H. (2018). A new inflammatory marker: elevated monocyte to HDL cholesterol ratio associated with smoking. *Journal of Clinical Medicine*, *7*(4), 76. https://doi.org/10.3390/jcm7040076

Young, E. (2013, February 25). *Neurons could outlive the bodies that contain them*. Science. https://www.nationalgeographic.com/science/article/neurons-could-outlive-the-bodies-that-contain-them

Youplushealth. (2020, August). *How to naturally boost human growth hormone (HGH)*. youplushealth. https://youplushealthusa.com/blog/how-to-naturally-boost-human-growth-hormone-hgh/

Zelman, K. M. (2008, February 21). *6 Steps to changing bad eating habits*. WebMD. https://www.webmd.com/diet/obesity/features/6-steps-to-changing-bad-eating-habits

Zeratsky, K. (2021, December 15). *HCG diet: is it safe and effective?* Mayo Clinic. https://www.mayoclinic.org/healthy-lifestyle/weight-loss/expert-answers/hcg-diet/faq-20058164#:~:text=Side%20effects%20have%20also%20been

Zhao, Y., Jia, M., Chen, W., & Liu, Z. (2022). The neuroprotective effects of intermittent fasting on brain aging and neurodegenerative diseases via regulating mitochondrial function. *Free Radical Biology and Medicine, 182*, 206–218. https://doi.org/10.1016/j.freeradbiomed.2022.02.021

Made in United States
Troutdale, OR
10/20/2023